Teresa Kay

PICK UR SMILE

Common Sense Dentistry

ISBN: 1475016158
ISBN-13: 9781475016154
Library of Congress Control Number: 2012904897
CreateSpace, North Charleston, South Carolina

Acknowledgment

Russ Hall, thanks for encouraging me,
to put thoughts to paper.

Don Smith thanks for your help in translating my
jumble into paragraphs.

My daughters and granddaughters, my love for you,
there are no words.

TK

Blessed by all the things, done right

Still ridden by all the things I wish I could redo

Through it all

I Like Myself

I Love My Life

TK

Contents

This book is in no way a diagnosis of any dental problems

This book is to be used to assist in the
Common Knowledge of Dentistry

If you think you need to see a Dentist,
You are months Past Due

We in the dental field are here to help and guide **you**

To a healthier and more functional smile

Pick UR smile

Many years of on-the-job training have provided me with a language and a few insights that make it easier for me to discuss dental problems in a more comprehensive and patient-friendly manner. This communication is beneficial to the health of patients who, after all, are the reason I receive a paycheck at the end of each month. Communication breaks down the barrier between what a doctor knows and what a patient understands. The following is the accumulation of information and knowledge received by many conversations. Thank you patients, for teaching me so much about the field, that I love working in.

After I had the first ten years under my belt, I made the bold statement that there was nothing else for me to learn; I believed I had seen it all. Then, at work one day, I stepped out to call in the next patient. A mother and daughter stepped forward to walk with me to the room. The daughter stopped, turned and pulled her gum out of her mouth, then placed it in her mother's mouth. "I want that back when we get to the car," she said. I never again will make the mistake of thinking I've seen everything.

ONE "MUST" QUESTION TO ASK:
Some states do not require that a dentist carry malpractice insurance. Asking about this insurance is a good question to review. Lawyers want to be paid for their service soon after the settlement, not wait on the dentist to sell property or other items to come up with the amount. Lawyers might not take your case if there is no insurance company to assure payment. If something goes wrong with a big case, you, the patient, might be out a lot of money. Dental professionals are just people who have read different books and are good with their hands in tight places. You might find yourself in a lot of discomfort, and incur more expense to stabilize and return the harmony to your facial muscular structure and tissue. If you do feel that your teeth are not clean when you leave the hygienist, please say so. This is no different then bringing home an article from the cleaners and it still has the stain. Be proactive in selection of a provider and product you receive just as any other purchase

This is a book about Common Sense Dentistry.

Why are dental procedures so expensive?

Dental work (the making of dentures, crowns and bridges) is done with many of the same steps with which fine jewelry is made. Artificial teeth that work with precision are custom-made jewelry for the mouth that must remain aesthetically attractive along with being compatible with oral tissue, withstanding temperature and PH changes and almost a thousand pounds of pressure that can be produced by the facial muscles during REM sleep (dream sleep). The nerve system will shut down the muscle pressure at around three hundred pounds-per-inch during the waking hours. (This is enough to crack pecans.) Patients are usually sorry that they did not take better care of their real teeth when they had the chance.

A universal truth is that in the medical field you should believe everything we tell you until we decide to change our mind. Research and development are an on going adventure in all fields of medicine, quit exciting. This is why you will find me in the hammock reading these magazines and books, I am quit the nerd.

IF YOUR WISH IS TO MAKE THE DENTAL PROFESSION AS PROFITABLE AS POSSIBLE TO ALL WHO ARE IN IT, HERE ARE SOME OF THE HABITS YOU CAN HAVE THAT WILL ENSURE THEY KEEP DRIVING A BETTER CAR THAN YOU:

Let's imagine for a moment that you are hungry. You take a walk into the kitchen, one that in this case is very dirty. Roaches are snacking on the Pop Tarts; ants are as thick as the spaghetti noodles; mice are swimming in the soda pop; snakes are tanning themselves on a peanut butter sandwich. Are you hungry now?

The proportional size of the undesirable critters is larger, but if you did not brush your teeth since the last meal that's how the inside of your mouth looks. Every breath you take brings in bacteria that think your mouth is no different than the kitchen I just described.

Parents often say, "I can't get the kids to brush." Tell them about that dirty kitchen. Not brushing is like not washing the dishes and leaving them on the table for the next meal. Tell them that not flossing is like not washing the silverware. That's a visual image that might stick.

Habits That Will Increase Your Dental Visits

SIP COKES ALL DAY (Light or dark color: if it bubbles when it is poured) (Dr Pepper, Sprite, Mt Due, Pepsi, Coca Cola or any other)

Your mouth works at a PH of around seven (7). Ask any mechanic how many times they have used cokes to clean metal. All types of cokes have a PH of less than two (2) in a can at room temperature. Over ice and through a straw this moves to an upper three (3) PH level. Car battery acid is one (1)! Google, food PH chart!

Have a contest with friends: see whose brand of coke will melt the penny first.

Place a penny in a cup

Replace fresh coke, any type, over the penny each day.

The penny will be gone in the fourteen to twenty day. That right, it will melt metal. Who will be the first to have a cavity? (Hint: The one at room temp)

NEVER EAT ICE CUBES, OTHER THAN SOFT SHAVED ICE
What happens to anything that is cold and slammed together?
Cracks and fractures, in general it breaks.
"But I was only eating an egg sandwich when half my tooth fell off!"
The tooth gave way at that time, but it fractured during the affair with ice!

EAT STICKY CANDY such as fruit roll up gummy bears, even raisins.

Adults know how some food stick to your teeth. Children's Teeth are softer by nature and will decay faster. Children have no desire to remove the good sweet taste. Bacteria are invited in with every breathe, for a free dinner. Cavity bugs food is carbs: a perfect sample is lodged between the teeth.

BE A GUM CHEWER The tooth surface has defects called pits and fissures. The sugar that makes the gum so tasty gets packed into these defects. (Sealants, which will be discussed later, contain components that plug these holes.) Xyilitol is a cavity retardant as it slows decay. Gums such as Spry, Orbit, and Trident contain this chemical, and are safer to chew. (Look for the ADA seal) Just because a gum's label says" Sugar Free" does not mean it will be "Cavity Free".
Chewing gum is like lifting weights to the facial muscles, and can lead to hammering down on the teeth with more force than the tooth can handle. Possibilities of fractured teeth and abscess could be in your future. So don't chew gum all day.

SNACK ON PROCESSED FOOD
This includes foods smashed or ground down to smaller partials, like chips, crackers, cereal and cookies. Processed food comes in pieces that are just the right size for feeding the bacteria that are in the air around us. The moisture in the mouth, along with the air we breathe, provides bacteria with the equivalent of a table, chairs, plates and maybe even napkins.

DRY MOUTH
This is the most destructive thing that can happen to teeth. Whole section is set aside for this problem. Check to see if your medication has this element as a side effect. Use a mouth moisturizing spray every hour, if needed.

Beneficial Habits That Can Help You Avoid Dental Visits

FLOSS THEN BRUSH, THEN CONTINUE ON THE TONGUE
You would clean out the corners of a room in your house before you sweep the room clean. The same goes for your mouth. Clean out between the teeth with floss, and then brush it all away. Brush your tongue too since it has a formation on the top that look like mushrooms. Food particles hide under the caps of these mushrooms and cause irritation. The tongue will also get upset with what is left behind and start changing colors, from white to tan, possibly even brown and black. Black hair on your tongue is one long-term possibility. This occurs when the surface of the tongue has a metamorphoses change into hair-like follicles. Oral surgeons will give your tongue a haircut and send you home after telling you to: "BRUSH YOUR TONGUE!" If this brushing motion gags you, stop and take a deep breath. Don't hold your breath while you are brushing your tongue. Holding your breath may activate your gag reflex.

WHEN FLOSSING
> Hold a short piece of floss between two fingers
>> On Each Side of a Tooth
> See-Saw the floss in a slow downward motion
>> There is a light contact between teeth
>> GENTLE slide the floss between tooth and gum
>> This is the area where the popcorn kernel hangs
>> Pull the floss into a 'C' shape on one side of tooth
>> Slide up and down a couple of times.
>> Repeat other side and all of the teeth.
> IT WILL BE SORE FOR, FIRST FOUR DAYS
> STOP FOR FOUR DAYS, BLEEDING START

> YOU-TUBE HAS LOTS OF DEMOS

Flossing

USE A CLEAN SEGMENT BETWEEN EACH TOOTH

All flossing does is place a piece of sting in a very tight space and scoops up junk.

Every breath you take in contains two kinds of bacteria. One is aerobic, meaning that it needs air. It sits on top of the tooth and eats the carbohydrates. Anything that eats has waste. Bacteria waste is very acidic like that can of soda, acid eats at the surface of the tooth. The result is a cavity. This bacteria does not have time to reproduce because it has to deal with the actions of the tongue, cheek and swallowing, unless you provide a hole, crack or space that will provide air.

The second type of bacteria is anaerobic meaning that it does not need air. It will hide in the flap of tissue between your gums and teeth, where the bits of popcorn kernels like to hide. For a while the bacteria will think only of itself, snacking on the food left between your teeth. But remember, anything that eats will reproduce and have waste. Soon there will be sisters, uncles, grandkids and cousins all living in the enclosed area. THE GANG WILL BE HUNGRY. There is just not enough food left between the teeth to feed this family reunion. They will start talking to each other: "See that pink piece of tissue between the teeth? As a gang we can produce the chemicals to turn that muscle into hamburger meat and as hamburger we can eat it."

Older people are often said to look "long in the tooth." The teeth did not move up. The bacteria ate its way down, consuming parts of the face. Yes, part of your facial structure!

When a thorn is in the skin too long the body will slowly package up the invader, move the problem up/out and you can just scratch it off. As the infection increases around the tooth the body will do whatever it can to protect the jaw bone. The problem is housed by the teeth. The body can't package up the tooth, so it removes the support holding the tooth in position. Sooner or later, the body will get rid of the problem tooth or teeth to save the face. Then a person's chin and nose will soon become close friends.

If your leg was bleeding!

Would you say you have taken a good bath?

When blood is spit out with tooth brushing!

We shrug it off and rinse.

NOTHING BLEEDS WHEN IT IS HEALTHY

BLOOD IS TOO PRECIOUS TO THE BODY

Just think of it as the blood that was feeding the bacteria. Now you have knocked some of them off with the toothbrush. They were sucking on you like a leech. This is a symptom of being sick, having a sore, or an infection.

You may see people with red halos around their teeth. Collectively they represent a sore about the size of a quarter. Purple or red areas in-between the teeth mean the sore is the size of the thumb and finger make a circle. Loose teeth or white patches between them mean the sore is as BIG as the palm of your hand. It's no wonder you want to step back from the breath of a people with this condition; that smell is pus.

Flossing is hard. It's like tying your shoe, on your tongue, backward, and in the dark. Use the "Easy Flossers" that are available and in most stores. Avoid the type that looks like a bow or horseshoe. They make it too hard to reach the back teeth. **Use the kind that looks like the fangs of a snake**. Your back teeth are your workhorses; give them special attention. Remember that floss scoops up bacteria. Don't help bacteria spread by using a short piece over and over. Use a fresh piece of string between each tooth. Take out about a yard of string floss or a dozen of the floss holders. They're cheap—DENTAL WORK IS NOT!

Toothpicks are excellent for after meals. Do not take the place of good home care.

Toothbrushes

GO FOR **SOFT** ONLY

"YOU ARE NOT CLEANING THE BBQ PIT"

SMALLER SIZES BRUSHES
   MOVES AROUND THE TEETH BETTER

The teeth should only be massaged in slow, small rotations. By taking a toothbrush to the TV, computer, or reading area and massaging the tissue and the teeth, it will make a big difference in the overall taste in your mouth. That's right, with a dry toothbrush slowing messaging the lovely smile, and fresh breath; you would like to share with others. Promise you'll replace your toothbrush every other month. Pick an even or odd month and walk through the house and replace all the brushes. Tooth brushes are cheap compared to dental work.

Toothbrushes do the same work as a wash cloth; you would not bathe with a month old wash cloth! Don't just smell your toothbrush before rinsing or applying the toothpaste, replace it before it sours.

You may say: "I like my hard brush and I feel it really gets the job done." Great, but keep in mind that it will cost over a thousand dollars per tooth to restore the enamel with a manmade, and lesser quality product.

How could a tooth brush do anything like that to your teeth?

Well, remember that water carved the Grand Canyon. Do something long enough and often enough, it will make a mark.

There are brushes on the market that are inches in length. Please reserve these and hard toothbrushes for your pets, household chores and removing wax from the groves of the car.

Teresa Kay

Electric toothbrushes are great, but you don't marry the brush head.

They may be more expensive than manual toothbrushes, but think about the wash cloth again. Change the brush head as often as you would your regular toothbrush. For anyone with hand-related disabilities, an electric version is a must. If a person has difficulty holding a pen, then consider that the toothbrush is close to the same size.

Any product that is added after flossing and brushing is of little assistance.

Flossing can cleans the largest percentage of the waste in your mouth. Brushing can clean the smaller percentage of the waste. NO MOUTH IS EVER STERILE!

JUST DON'T MARRY THE BRUSH
REPLACE IT OFTEN.

YOU MIGHT NOT BE ABLE TO RECOVER FROM THAT COLD OR FLU BECAUSE IT IS ON THE TOOTHBRUSH. YOU KEEP GIVING IT BACK TO YOUSELF.

TEETH SHOULD NOT BE WEARING SWEATER TO BED. LET THE TONGUE SLIDE ACROSS YOUR TEETH AND KEEP BRUSHING OR FLOSSING UNTIL THEY FEEL SMOOTH AND SLICK!

Toothpaste

Use whatever brand you like. Fluoride is the best chemical in toothpaste. Since its introduction, dental cavities have been greatly reduced. If you have trouble with sensitivity to cold this could be your hero. Fluoride takes twenty minutes to do its work and it is water soluble. When you rinse out your mouth ALL of the chemicals you paid for just went down the drain.

When the foam fills your mouth, use it as a mouth wash. HOLD it for a minute, then spit and walk away. Fluoride is a free radical and needs time to bind and mend damaged areas. (I'll be covering this again in the sensitive teeth section)

What kind of active ingredient in toothpastes should you consider?

There are three kinds:
    Stannous fluoride
    Potassium fluoride
    Sodium fluoride

What taste do you like, and which one helps with your sensitivity?

Sensitive toothpaste has two of the above chemicals.

If sensitivity does not improve in 7 to 10 days, change types of fluoride.

It is listed as an active ingredient on the toothpaste's box.

The percentage of whitening chemical is not strong enough to do much except remove the stain that was placed on the teeth that day.

The tarter control is an excellent chemical, but be careful. It might be the reason for the irritation to the tissue in your mouth. It may even cause peeling of that tissue.

Plain baking soda is good for removing day-to-day stains. Just place a small amount in the palm of your hand and Brush Gently. Follow up with fluoride toothpaste. Remember if a food or drink has color it has the possibility of staining your teeth.

You need fluoride.

Tobacco stain is an aromatic stain that permeates the tooth and is a great deal harder to remove. You need more powerful chemicals, like the ones found in the tooth whitening compounds in dental offices.

Fluoride

Here is a chemical that needs to be added to your nightly routine at every age. Fluoride is not just for children. With our diets having so much processed food and carbonated drinks (cokes), the cavity years just don't seem to stop. Mature adults have the added occurrence of recession. This is where the nice warm 98 degree tissue around the tooth just scoots down, exposing more of the tooth surface. This area has not had the advantage of daily exposure to toothpaste and is not as strong as the enamel or crown part of the tooth.

Fluoride is not the only element need to complete the repair need for teeth. Calcium and phosphate need to be present in the diet and saliva for a complete reaction to happen on the tooth. These compounds are present in vitamins and a diet with daily dairy (calcium). Phosphate is found in fruits, nuts, whole grain, leafy vegetables, meats, and dairy products.

Fluoride should be applied on all the surfaces that have a portion of a partial surrounding them. This clap will add to the presents of food being held against the tooth surface. Place a small toothbrush into the opening of the missing tooth and message the side of the tooth and apply fluoride nightly. This also holds true for the appliances use in braces.

Fluoride will also assist in the protection of teeth when you have a dry mouth. The saliva rinses and adds a protective enzyme army to the teeth. If the elements in saliva are reduced, you will do yourself a world of good to apply Fluoride nightly. When beaching teeth, fluoride will be necessity.

Fluoride is the hero when there is the discomfort from cold articles in the mouth. If ice in your drink or enjoying a nice crisp salad hurts your teeth; use fluoride.

THERE ARE THREE KINDS:
>Stannous fluoride
>Potassium fluoride
>Sodium fluoride

You will have to find the one that best suits your body chemistry and diet.

Look for "Active Ingredient" on the content labels.

Bleaching

Bleaching cleans out the pores of the tooth with a bubbling action. The question of whether it causes damage is still under investigation. There are some studies that say it benefits the tissue with oxygen exchange. I just keep reading.

Do you know any middle-aged person whose teeth look as if they ate rocks, all chipped and jagged? That person had chalk white teeth in high school—the kind everyone is dying to have. The calcium has a shorter shelf life than any of the other components of the tooth structure. Look around at all the older people who still have strong, useable teeth they are yellow or gray. The yellow tooth has the best success in the chemical warfare of bleaching and will not lose its duration strength. Gray will become whiter, but not reach the color most people are trying to obtain.

The tooth has pores just like the skin and the hydrogen peroxide that is used to whiten teeth is no different than the brown bottle that you see sitting around the house, just stronger. The brown bottle is only 2 percent; the strips and boxes that can be picked up at the local stores are up to around 10 percent. Dental offices can dispense hydrogen peroxide in ranges up to thirty percent. They all work; it just depends on how much time and money you want to spend. Over the counter treatments take about ten to fourteen days and have to be repeated every three to four months. Boxes will cost at or above twenty dollars. Also watch expiration dates and don't think you can save a few doses for the next round of whitening. That's about a hundred to a hundred and fifty dollars a year, after year, after year. Bleaching teeth is like coloring your hair: it has to be repeated, and maintained.

If your teeth are cold sensitive, place the bleaching chemical on the teeth for a short period of time, 5 minutes, wait till the next day to see if your reaction is desirable. When bleaching was in its early years the chemicals were different and they made MY teeth hurt for the entire night.

A dental office supply of whitener can amount to a couple of hundred dollars, for the take-home tray kit. The time you spend bleaching is seven to ten days. Bleach as much as you want, but the best effect is seen in the first two days. Recommended time is ten to fourteen days. Be smart and look at the teeth that are stubborn to change and only place chemical on that tooth in your custom trays for a couple of days, till the stubborn tooth matches the other teeth. Then return to bleaching them all, but stop after fourteen days. Not all of us can have Chiclets for teeth. In about twenty minutes, the chemicals have done their thing. Keeping the trays in any longer is just going to do fine tuning in the angles. Manufacture recommendation is one hour.. DO NOT GO SLAM DUNK A COLD DRINK AFTER THIS. THERE IS A CHANCE YOU WILL CRY. COLD SENSITIVITY IS THE BIGGEST SIDE EFFECT OF BLEACHING. The chemical reaction of bleaching dries the teeth out, and it takes the body over three days to rehydrate.

Refill kits are about ten to fifteen dollars for another tube (sold in sets of 4 to 8). At that price, with only bleaching after cleanings, bleaching about every other month and on special occasions, custom version from the dental offices will be cheaper in the long run. Watch for dental office specials, which usually run during holidays such as Christmas and Valentine's Day.

In-office bleaching, means the use of stronger chemical under supervision with the ability to have the fourteen day chemical reaction occur in a couple of hours. Some of the chemicals need a light for reaction to happen. Some just need time and stirring. Do remember the sensitivity to cold. In office cost will generally include the take home trays and chemical for you to maintain your sparkle.

IF YOU CAN TASTE THE CHEMICALS YOU ARE WASTING THE CHEMICALS, (in your take home trays). Just place a small dab (about the size of pencil lead) in the tray. Store your trays and chemicals in the fridge. Do not take custom trays in hot cars, as they may melt.

Mouthwashes

DID YOUR CAR EVER COME CLEAN BY SPRAYING IT WITH THE GARDEN HOSE AND NOT SCRUBBING? You will remove the dust, but very little of the road grime. Generally, it takes a little bit of elbow grease and rubbing. The damage to our teeth is caused by a sticky component that is hard to remove because it has to deal with the motion of our lips, cheeks and tongue. This is no easy environment to live around in the mouth, but through the year's bacteria has learned how to hide and make a home.

A mouthwash only works while you taste it. Swishing it over the top of the bacteria's home on your tooth does little to the apartment complex under development there. Just removes the dust. With every breath you will be replacing the cluster of organism just eliminated. The working chemical is alcohol in around thirty percent of big name products. Beer and wine by comparison contain around ten percent alcohol and you need a license to sell them.

Overuse of any chemical will cause a burn and the gums will peel like the skin does when sunburned. Mouth rinses dry the mouth and can cause peeling.

Also, there may be white, stringy, movable pieces. This is similar to and can be confused with cancer in stage one.

Breath mints (now here is a money-maker for the dentist) let sugar rest on your teeth. Sugar-free does not mean cavity-free. Keep the majority of the food off your teeth and the bacteria will not have a café to eat at, nor will they generate a waste that causes the breath you do not want anyone to smell.

Dry Mouth

ONE OF THE MOST DESTRUCTIVE
OCCURANCE IN THE MOUTH
(In my opinion)

Enzymes swim in our saliva. They kill a great deal of the bacteria that come into the mouth with every breath (Just imagine them as the football team at the pizza parlor after the Friday night game.)   As bacteria enters the mouth, these enzymes gobble up undesirable components and shield /protect the teeth.

Under the tongue and on the cheek are glands for the production of fluid that keep the mouth moist. The enzymes survive and thrive in this liquid. Loss of this moisture will happen to almost everybody as the birthdays start totaling up. When these enzymes are reduced, or missing, the teeth lose the strongest army they have in their fight against decay, and you also lose stage one in the digestion of food.

A patient came into one of the dental offices where I worked. They had done all the right things for their children's dental health. The kids had moved on in their lives, and it was time for the parent to indulge in a smile for which they had always hoped and dreamed; so all the teeth were crowned. Within months of the completion of the new smile, there was a development: big health problems and they were told to take medication every day, for the rest of their life.

OF THE TOP FOUR HUNDRED PRESCRIBED MEDICATION, THREE HUNDRED AND EIGHTY OF THEM HAVE A SIDE EFFECT THAT COULD CAUSE DRY MOUTH IN MANY INDIVIDUALS.

Read labels!

This very nice person moved before the next regular check-up time came around at the dentist who provided all of this lovely dental work. The person did not find a new dentist for almost a year and a half, yet, followed all the instruction provided by the dental staff, and keep their mouth very clean. But without the enzymes, "dry" mouth had destroyed everything: decay was present on almost every side of every crown in their mouth. Ten's of thousands of dollars worth of work was coming apart with decay, as there is only a small part of the natural tooth under the crown that secures the crown to the root/jaw bone. This is the only part left to decay. When this portion of the tooth is weak or damaged, there is nothing to keep the crown glued to your smile.

There are a couple of over-the-counter treatments for dry mouth. These are easy to find at any supermarket or pharmacy. Biotene is the oldest product on the market and the companies will mail you samples for free. I like and use the 'Moisturizing Spray or Gel'. If the taste isn't to your satisfaction, there are other similar products available. Use the product every hour, if need be. At bedtime every night and if you wake up in the nights, use the moisturing sprays. It is cheap; dental work is not. If your tongue feels dry or sticky, or you hear a click of the tongue when speaking, use something. Water will reduce the dryness, but will not provide the necessary enzymes.

Radiation treatment around the head and neck also lead to destruction of the saliva glands which make the moisture. This is common knowledge. As part of the rehab treatment fluoride trays and dry mouth chemicals are commonly used. Discussion with the cancer specialist is becoming standard of care in the recovery treatment of cancer.

Be a commander of your own health. With all the information available about medications and treatments, search out all you can, and inform yourself before side effects lead to bigger and more destructive events in your life.

This is a book about Common Sense Dentistry

Treatment Received In A Dental Office And What To Expect

Pre-Med

Patients are often asked to take four tablets
before dental treatment.

So many questions are raised about this procedure.

Now if you had a choice of swallowing a couple of pills or returning to surgery for the removal and replacement of your joint implant, what is your choice?

Sure, there is a chance the meds might upset your stomach or give you a yeast infection. This can be resolved by eating yogurt **ONE** hour after taking the tablets. In fact, after all antibiotics, yogurts will assist in replacing the elements essential in the digestive track to absorb the minerals and vitamins the body needs. Antibiotic's attack all bacteria within its capabilities; ugly, bad and those that are needed. This will explain why long term use of antibiotics will give you the runs; things are running a muck in your regular digestive function. **No** yogurt along with the antibiotic tablets, at the same time, the two will just work on each other and have no benefit to your problem or health. There are tablets that can be chewed that have the same compound: ask the pharmacist.

Exams By The Dentists

Lawsuits changes the style in which the medical field practices.

Standard of care must met or exceed the needs of the patient in order to protect the license that your professional is working under.

Don't say "I WOULDN'T SUE "

The thought has passed through everyone's mind.

Limited Exam — **One** tooth and **one** problem only (x-rays and evaluation)

You are limited to that tooth in the mouth and no other problems can be discussed at that visit or on a phone call. **You requested limits**.

Comprehensive Exam — Evaluation of **all** hard and soft tissue of the mouth

Includes an Oral Cancer Exam   Problems that arise in the **near** future can be discussed with other member of the dental team without an appointment with the doctor. (Note the work NEAR) Cost is not that much more than a Limited Exam

Periodic Exam   **Regular** visit with Dentist yearly

Most states require yearly x-rays as Standard of Care.

Reading of the X-rays, Oral Cancer Exam, Cavity evaluation,

Perio evaluation (how the teeth and gums are getting along)

Review patients question and health history update

Oral Cancer Exam

DON'T THINK CANCER IS ONE COLOR
ONE SIZE OR SHAPE
NORMAL IS BILATERAL (same on both sides)
SORE AND/ OR INFECTION SHOULD HEAL IN
2 WEEKS, in the mouth
ANYTHING THAT TAKES LONGER

NEEDS TO BE SEEN BY A DOCTOR
Abnormalities need to be evaluated by a
Specialist in the medical field

Exception: Geographic Tongue
(patterns on the tongue change about monthly)

Oral cancer exam might be preformed by other staff members and/or the doctor.

Findings are review with the doctor and they will frequently repeat similar steps. The doctor will take all necessary step needed in referral or answering questions and concerns. Don't be alarmed of you are ask to return in two week to have the area reviewed by the doctor, or if photos are taken for reference. Occurrences of head and neck cancer seem to be on the rise and your best interest is always first in your doctor's procedures. Better Safe than Sorry.

Steps in a Visual Oral Cancer Exam

This is A method of performing an Oral Cancer Exam.

Gloved hand
    View the roof of the mouth
    Touch the tongue to the roof of the mouth
        Under the tongue; both sides should match
    View of the tonsil area
        Please relax your tongue; give us a view
    Hold the tongue with dry gauze;
        Both sides of the tongue should match
    Place a finger under the tongue and one in the
        chin area Check for lumps.
    Close teeth –Pull out lips and view area
        between cheek/lips and teeth.

Take off the gloves
    Moving hands in a smooth motion equally
        on the sides of the face, along chin
    Chin to Neck-both sides should feel the same
    Neck to Shoulders-both sides should feel the same
    Swallow the Thyroid should feel
        like the shape of a heart
    Back of Neck in the area of the Hair line
        Take your time there a many Nodes
            in this area, from the sinuses
            In fact this is the nice part,
            providing the patient with a message.
    Squeeze the sides of the Neck (gentle)
        Question: Is this sore or tender?

Doctor will review and/or repeat many of these steps, during their exam.

X-Rays (Radiographs)

X-Rays give the Doctor a big chunk of the visual that guides treatment.

The film must be placed in an area that provides the best view of the infected area. I know you are hurting and you are asking to bite on the same tooth that keeps you up all night. With out a correct view to see the infection no treatment can be provided. Often you will find you will be referred out, to more expense and another x-ray, if a clear view can not be provide for doctor.

SO HOLD STILL,
DON'T MOVE THE FILM
GIVE US A BREAK
X RAY FILMS ARE; ONE SIZE FITS NO ONE
THE STAFF IS TRYING TO DO THEIR JOB
IF THEY MISS THE VIEW THE DOCTOR WILL SEND THEM
BACK TO HURT THE SAME AREA AGAIN UNTIL THE
PROBLEM CAN BE DETECTED AND A VIEW IS PROVIDED
FOR SOLID TREATMENT PROOF.

There are slight shades of gray and black that are present on the films.

The white area is metal present in the mouth.

Metal fillings and crowns show up as a big white area.

The white/light grayish is the shell of enamel that is visible in the mouth

Also the shade of tooth color fillings

The light gray is the dentin of the tooth and is weaker than enamel or the tooth

Dentinal tubules house the nerve that cause the cold discomfort

The light gray line in the middle of the tooth is the nerve/blood supply, housing.

The light charcoal with whitish webbing is the jaw bone, (air holes), so our skinny little neck can hole up our cannonball size head.

The darkest blacks to charcoal areas are the sinuses cavities. They will look whitish if the area is filled with fluid. (It will be drain out your nose soon)

Cleaning (Prophy)

(There are three different types)

I Regular Cleaning

Even with the best of home care, no one can clean every angle, groove, pit, and stain out of their mouth on a daily basis. So for this reason alone, go to the dental office. With the use of a bright light they will have a straight on view, and shine up your smile. You should be offered a pair of glasses to shield your eyes from the flying toothpaste. Shades would be nice to reduce the glare of the bright light. But the most important activity of the visit should be the education about the areas missed, with home care information and tools to assist you in the new goal of home care. The gold star of the visit is showing you the feeling of an accurate flossing.

GUM DISEASE (long in the tooth)

Treatment can only be successful with regular home care, diet changes, and commitment

With every breath two kinds of bacteria enter the mouth. Do not worry; they have been there for countless years and do little harm. We really need them for some of the digestive functions.

One of the types of bacteria needs air, (aerobic) and sits on top of the tooth eating carbohydrates. Their acid waste will cause cavities. Anything that eats has waste and this waste material is very acidic and etches a hole in the tooth. That means cavities.

Another type of bacteria that rides in with every breath does not need air (anaerobic). This bacterium will find the area where all the popcorn kernels also seem to have a homing device, and settle in rent free; the space between tooth and gum. Upon entering the flap of tissue, the organism will fight for survival, self- replicate (start a family), and of course produce waste. Anything that eats has waste. The nice pink tissue that forms the triangle between teeth is a muscle, as tough as steak. The waste formed by bacteria hiding in that flap of tissue will break up the muscle as if it were sent through a grinder to make hamburger meat. WHY? Because the bacteria can now eat this meat and use the blood supply as a source of food.

Teeth are not directly connected to the jaw bone. Both are bone surfaces and would rub each other to oblivion, just like two pieces of chalk. There is a space between the tooth and jaw bone called a Periodontal Ligament. It acts like a shock absorber and cushions the movement of the tooth during chewing. Want to feel one of them right now? Just take a bite of roast beef or chicken! The reason the stuff packs between your teeth is the movement of these ligaments. One side of the tooth is smashed and the other side is stretched. Take the food item out and the tooth will stabilize itself and comfort will return. This collar around the tooth where the popcorn kernels hide provides a breading ground for bacteria.

Wonder why you have to take a premeditation of an antibiotic before a dental appointment sometimes? It is because there is a chance that the bacteria that live in even the healthiest of mouths will be introduced to the blood stream and cause damage to other organs just as it has been doing in the mouth.

These are just a few common sense observation collected from patients statements

Doctors noticed a high likelihood of gum disease in some types of sick patients, which were just slow to recover for treatment. Studies are available to show that healing tissue will be affected by poor dental home care and bleeding gums. This is why patients need full dental tissue evaluation these days before they can receive a lung transplant, heart, or undergo other invasive surgeries. All joint implants are suggested to be premedicated with say, Penicillin or a similar medication for the same reason. Would you rather swallow a couple of pills or have your knee implant region swell twice to it size. It can happen. This is also why, for people with gum disease, arthritis might be more intense.

THAT POTTY MOUTH HAS A FULL BODY EFFECT.
- THE HEAD BONE IS CONNECTED TO THE NECK BONE
- THE NECK BONE IS CONNECTED TO THE SHOULDER BONE
- THE INFECTED JAW BONE JUST MIGHT BE THE REASON FOR THE HEART ATTACK

Flossing

Take a little piece of string and slid it between the teeth, with a gentle sawing motion, pull a C-shape toward both side of the space, move up and down a few times. Do this to all the spaces between your teeth, and do it every day until there is no bleeding. Stop flossing the day you wish to increase your chances of wearing dentures. People who are smokers may not even get the warning of bleeding because the tissue is cauterized (slightly cooked) by heat.

II Debridement

The removal of the top layer of buildup

Have you ever tried to remove a thorn from your hand? You dig and dig then there comes a time when you have had enough, but you still see some of the thorn in the area. You wait a few days, maybe a week, start removing more of the thorn, but now there is not as much discomfort since the body was given the time to stabilize the good tissue. Wait long enough and the body will package together the remaining portion of the thorn, and push it to the surface to be scratched off. This is what will happen in the mouth if the top layer of tarter and plaque is removed, the tissue around the tooth will heal a bit. Every bit of tissue counts. Any that is lost is gone forever. Oral tissue will not grow back if it is removed by the bacteria or with the treatment provided.

So let the tissue heal for a week to ten days, after the first cleaning. Return to the dental office to allow the hygienist finish the job by fine tuning the surface of the teeth. Have you ever been so dirt that you hosed off first outside before you took a shower?

III Scale and Root Plane

A deeper cleaning

The dentist will come in and numb the mouth just as they would if you were having a filling. Generally half of the mouth will be done at two separate visits no more that 14 days apart. (Could be made into four appointment but remember the 14 days over all, needs to be considered). No longer, the first parts of healing tissue will be contaminated by the other sides; because you are eating and breathing. This type of cleaning is to remove waste that has taken up residence deep in the tissue and is mounted to the tooth.

Bacteria have settled in for the long haul (building condos, shopping centers and recreational facilities); reinforcement must be sent into the side of the tooth to create a stronger structure, to assure longevity. Just removing the organism that is present in the flap of tissue and on the side of the tooth will not complete the job. The tissue will move back to rest on the surface of the tooth and find the villains still living in the tooth. There the tissue will find the waste products and back away from a former enemy. This deep cleaning removes a sliver on the side of the tooth: it is like mowing down a neighborhood to the growing bacterial enemy and removes most of the reinforcement the bacteria sent into the tooth structure.

In general, people will return to the 'old home care habits' and in two years time this type of deep cleaning will need to be repeated. You have allowed a bad type of bacteria to make such a residence in you mouth, it will take over a year for change to occur and the mouth return back to normal flora.

NO MOUTH IS STERILE

Yep, some things just need repeated.

Flossing

Take a little piece of string and slid it between the teeth, with a gentle sawing motion, pull a C-shape toward both side of the space, move up and down a few times. Do this to all the spaces between your teeth, and do it every day until there is no bleeding. Stop flossing the day you wish to increase your chances of wearing dentures. People who are smokers may not even get the warning of bleeding because the tissue is cauterized (slightly cooked) by heat.

Sealants

A tooth is made up of seeds that fuse together in the face, as the body develops. This is why the young front teeth have ridges, those funny half circles on the edge. They are gone all too soon because the tongue likes to polish smooth everything within its reach. That's what happens to a chipped tooth as well. Just chip a tooth anywhere and the tongue will polish that spot smooth, right after it has caused a sore and maybe an ulcer on the tongue.

The back teeth are made of four seeds: the four corners of the molars. As these teeth fuse during formation, there can be mistakes called pit and fissures (holes and lines). A sealant material can be flowed into these voids to assist in the prevention of cavities. Without the sealant it is nearly impossible to keep such a pit clean. A single toothbrush's fiber is often bigger than the pits: like a fist trying to clean out a donut hole.

Getting a sealant applied is affordable. Most insurance companies will pay 100% of the cost of having sealants applied because they know this prevents future cavities and is hence a good deal. From a parent's point of view, the process may also save a child sleepless nights due to dental pain. Even if the parent has to pay the full cost: it will be less than your portion left by the insurance company after a cavity is repaired, if a cavity forms.

When the sealants are finished and you sit up to leave, make sure the way your teeth come together and feels the same as it did when you arrived. Sometimes slight adjustments are needed to remove the sealant material from an area where it might have flowed on too thick. The difference of a width of hair can make the jaw muscles sore for a couple of days. You will chew or hit on the area enough to return it to the original position, but the professional can prevent this with just a mark of blue paper and tap of a dental instrument that removes just the excess sealant material.

Sealants reduce in the occurrences of decay on the top of the tooth.

SEALANTS
DO NOT
ASSIST IN
PREVENTION OF
CAVITIES
BETWEEN TEETH

EATING ICE
OR
HARD CANDY
CAN CHIP THE MATERIAL OUT
OF THE TOOTH

Dentists have a license: DDS- Doctor of Dental Surgery. Please note that the word Surgery is in the title. This is not a word to be taken lightly. Surgery means the work that will be provided with the use of local anesthesia. Other chemicals can be provided for the temporary assists with anxiety

Toothaches

You may say, "It doesn't hurt. I just catch food in the hole." Or, "I have saved myself so much money. I have not been to the dentist in years."

Thanks you, from all of us in the dental field, because when you do come in, you will spend **so much more** money that what you would have paid. A couple hundred dollars filling is now a couple thousand dollar root canal, with a build up and a crown. You're being foolish if you think this is a way to save.

When heat and pressure bother a tooth, the nerve inside has been compromised. That is going to make a tooth ache.

"Why? Can't the dentist just fill the hole with the filling stuff?"
It's like putting a top on a volcano!   **It will blow**.

With an infected tooth, the bacteria do not have to wait until you eat to have a meal. The main course is now your blood, tissue and nerve supply. Bacteria in the center of the tooth have a 24 hour food supply and 24 hours of waste. This waste not only goes into the mouth, some excess goes directly into your bloodstream. Have you ever seen someone's face swell up on one side, completely disfiguring it? Bacteria are going after the blood supply, bone and muscle of the face.

Look up the cause of death of the famous; Lucy, she has been on exhibit in many of the world big museums. Best bones are found in river beds, because the individual was there placing cold water on their hot, swollen face.

Medical Emergency team can only provide temporary relief. Pain will return.

Management And Anesthesia;

Behavioral Management:

Tooth structures are a very hard material. Teeth have to be, handling all the items that are placed in there for nutrition and habits. When repair is needed the instruments will be sharp, moving at a very high speed, and soft tissue can be harmed. Keeping still so that the procedure can be completed quickly, efficiently and safely, is critical. If extra hands, personnel or articles are needed there might be a charge. Quite often there is a referral to specialist. Repair of a very sick tooth could save your child sleepless nights and improve their health

Anesthesia:

Dentistry is a better world with chemistry. In very few events in life does someone get in your face, place their hands all over you and leave you numb.

With the introduction of the breathable gas nitrous, a patient can be placed in a semi-conscious state and leave with little side effect. Just make sure you are left on pure oxygen for ten minutes and allowed to set up and or stand up without being dizzy.

N2O: (Nitrous oxide) Breathable gas that will provide a feeling of light sleep. It is charge by the minute or hours. This is not a cheap drug. The person that is sitting in the room must have a license to even be there when the doctor has stepped out.

Painful Dentistry

Have you heard someone say, "This dentist just went ahead with the work and I felt it all"? They told the dentist to continue, they could not financial return.

The reason is the same as trying to mix water with oil. The medication used by dentists is thin like water. The infection (waste and bacteria) is thick like oil. Pus! Medication must be placed near the nerve supply, and the reason the patient is hurting is because the bacteria and its waste are on the nerve supply. The acidity of the infection also effects the medication: the drug simply can not reach the nerve ending. The more medication you take to stop the pain and prolonging having treatment, the only bacteria left after each prescription is the Superman version. This pus can be a thick as grease or lard. That's why the pain returns faster and more intensely, you are not taking care of the real problem, a hole in the tooth.

Most of the discomfort is caused by the swelling. Medication can reduce the pain from pressure. Reducing the swelling can give you minimal relief. Pain medications work on the information coming in to the brain, not in the area of the problem.

If you say, "Just pull the tooth. I have many others." Guess where every corn chip and sharp object is going to land for the rest of your life.

People that work at the liquor store <u>can not</u> help you. You will be just postponing the problems and allowing the Superman version of the bacteria to have another day to beat up and overcome the Nerd version of bacteria.

Yep! Just trying to teach you a little common sense to keep you out of needless

PAIN AND SLEEPLESS NIGHTS.

Fillings (Composite)

TOOTH-COLORED MATERIAL THAT HELPS FILL THE VOID OR CAVITIES

The tooth has six sides to it, like a box.
1. Front: mesial, toward the lips or center of the face
2. Back: distal, closes to the tonsils
3. Inside by the tongue: lingual
4. Cheek side: buccal for back teeth and facial for front teeth
5. Occulsal: top of the tooth or biting surface
6. Root of the tooth, buried in tissue and jawbone

The tooth will work the best through its life if it is left in its original whole structure. When decay eats a hole in the tooth, material must be placed into that hole that has the same strength, flexibility, agree with the tissue, and is easy working for the dentist.

The first step is to remove all of the active disease. The bacteria have been using your tooth as a dinner plate with an acidity level close to battery acid. The destruction of the tooth was just a side effect of bad table manners. Anything that eats has waste.

Bacteria come in with every breath and search for food that is left behind after a meal. NO MOUTH IS STERILE. These aerobic bacteria need air and a place to sit. (Any place will do: tartar, stains, cracks). Here the bacteria eat and produce waste that is very acidic. The structure of the tooth just breaks down and falls off. "Yeah," say the bacteria, "Now there is a couch and a reclining chair for my family. Because I am eating so well, I think I'll have a family now and start inviting a couple of the folks I see floating by. YEAH, now we have a shopping mall food court, entertainment center and better sleeping quarters. Keep it up for a couple of years and we'll have a water park and carnival."

After the filling is completed, just make sure that when the doctor is finished with the filling and sits you up that you can FLOSS the area and not have a spot that tears or hangs up the floss. This is called an overhang, or open margin. This will be a defect and allow a hiding hole for more bacteria to cause damage. The next cavity will be so close to the nerve supply it will increase the chances for a root canal and more than likely a crown. This defect is comparable to buying a set of tires and having the installer slit the tire half way through. It will function, but will not last as long as it's supposed to last. Floss should **GENTLY** be sawed between the teeth and glide down to the junction with the tissue. Pull the floss in to a C-shape, and then glide it freely to the area where it pops out, without a snag or fraying of the floss.

Decay can come very close to the nerve of the tooth but not enter the nerve chamber. Chemicals can be applied to the bottom of the drilled area, by the dentist, to stimulate a natural body function. As decay eats into the tooth center the body will notice the incoming attack and send out a message for the retreat of the nerve and blood supply. Bone will be laid by the surrounding cells to insulate the nerve. There is a dental chemical to stimulate this natural body function. If, after a filling, the tooth hurts but feels better as days pass, it's normal. If the discomfort stays the same, increases, or if heat hurts the tooth after a week, call the dentist's office. You waited too long to have the tooth filled and the nerve is mad. . Also, call the office if you feel the repaired tooth hitting first when you close your mouth. The long term effect of this could lead to damage of the nerve and could cause the need more extensive and expensive treatment, (like a stone bruise to the jaw bone), or could cause a break in the tooth.

Remember, doctors are just people who have read different books and can work in very small spaces. Your bite can change for

<u>laying down to sitting up</u>. Your mouth is numb and you are ask, to tap a couple of time, it might just be feeling better; but not just right. There is NO dental office without patients who are satisfied and tell others. Be proactive in seeking the best results from the service provided.

FILLINGS (composites) generally GROW UP TO BE CROWNS

Fillings are designed to last a dozen or more years
WITH
GOOD ORAL CARE AND HABIT

Crowns

A crown is like a thimble, covering the thumb to provide protection during uses. The tooth is cut back to remove either decay or defect, such as cracks and a shield is slid over the remaining portion of the tooth; must met the original design and shape of the tooth.

With the tooth under such pressure during usage (300 PSI while awake), it is hard for the remaining parts of a chipped tooth to hold the pieces together once the design is compromised.

When three or four-side are destroyed for any reason, discuss the options of a crown

The tooth has six sides to it, like a box.

1. Front: mesial, toward the lips or center of the face
2. Back: distal, closes to the tonsils
3. Inside by the tongue: lingual
4. Cheek side: buccal for back teeth and facial for front teeth
5. Occulsal: top of the tooth or biting surface
6. Root of the tooth, buried in tissue and jawbone

The tooth will work best through life if it is left in a whole piece. The more the sides of a tooth are destroyed, the more it needs coverage (something to hold the parts together) and not just repair. I have heard patients say "Just fill the thing." Dentists often reply, "I will guarantee the work to the parking lot." As with anything in nature, once a tooth is fractured by any defect, the whole structure will lose its overall original strength. Even a small filling could cause future problems.

If you wanted to split a log, you would place a wedge in the middle and hammer down on the top. A filling, whether tooth-colored or metal, will act like a log splitting wedge as you press down on the food you eat. It <u>could</u> increase the pressure in the filling or tooth, and the results could be a fracture. Drinking soda will destroy the tooth part of the filling in just a couple of years. The acid will find a happy home in the tiny, tiny space between the filling and the natural tooth and destroy the tooth. Don't worry; the filling will be in good shape, often falling out in your hand in just the shape it was in when the dentist placed it in your mouth. Just think of the dental office every time you pour that bubbly drink, when can I visit them next!

The crown is like a thimble over the pieces of the tooth: used to hold the tooth together. The crown is a manufactured substance that cannot get a cavity. The area under the crown where it meets the natural structure is still part of your body and needs TLC. This ledge area of the tooth is the most common area for failure. It is almost impossible to fill in the decay that is more than likely to have moved under the crown. The most common next step to occur is the purchase of a new crown.

FLOSS! –It's the only action that cares for a crown.

After the crown is completed, just make sure that when the doctor is finished with the crown and sits you up that you can FLOSS the area and not have a spot that tears or hangs up the floss. This is called an overhang, or open margin. This will be a defect and allow a hiding hole for more bacteria to cause damage. The next cavity will be so close to the nerve supply it will increase the chances for a root canal. This defect is comparable to buying a set of tires and having the installer slit the tire half way through. It will function, but will not last as long as it's supposed to last. Floss should **GENTLY** be sawed between the teeth and glide down to the junction with the tissue. Pull the floss in to a C-shape, and then glide it freely to the area where it pops out, without a snag or fraying of the floss.

Inlay/Onlay

A type of crown that fits into the prepared void of the tooth, or in and over the surfaces of the tooth. This method is chosen, to SAVE a much of the natural tooth structure or design as possible. (Natural tooth do have the stronger design.)

Veneers

These are like false finger nails.
Custom made porcelain chips, any shade of white.
Very delicate, produces a beautiful smile, saves tooth structure
Last ten of so years before edges can pickup stain or chip

Labial Veneer chair side: Eat an elbow, walk into a baseball or kiss the bottom of a swimming pool, just as I did. This is a quick fix. Don't trick your self into believing that this chemical can be used for all the functions that a natural tooth can perform. No heavy pressure should be applied to the edge of the filling, or you will have it in your hand or stomach real quick.

Veneer: The people that have the false fingers nail will truly understand this product. A custom make chip produced to fit over your own natural structure to assist in changing the color, and/or shape of your tooth. Generally cost is the same as a full crown but, you get to save your own natural strong tooth. This product will chip, and/or pop off, just like the fingernail product does. It is simply glued to a roughen surface of your tooth.

YOU MUST BE AWARE OF HOW YOU BITE INTO FOOD AND NEVER USE THEM TO OPEN UP EVEN A BOBBY-PIN OR BITE A FINGERNAIL, UNLESS YOU WANT NEW ONES.

Buildups On Crowns

Why does a crown need a buildup and what does this charge mean in my bill?

Placing a lid on the trashcan will not stop the smell and the things growing within.

Micro-leakage happens around almost all fillings within a couple of years, or a whole lot sooner if you do not have good home care, or if the crown fits poorly. This means that a space appears between the dental material and the natural tooth. The space can be so small that only a microscope can see the defects. Openings like this, though, are as large as the Brooklyn Bridge to bacteria.

A healthy surface must be designed under the crown. All of the natural tooth structure under the crown will be sealed away from detect for hopefully twenty years, the normal life span of crowns; the possibility of decay does not go away unless you floss correctly every day.

X-Rays will only show very large areas of destruction.

Flossing is the only thing that will clean and care for the supporting tooth structure.

Remember that it is not just the chicken and roast beef that packs between your teeth. Most of the crown area normally cleaned by a toothbrush is already designed not to decay. Message the edges with a brush and flossing between the teeth, where you're most likely to have problems.

Bridges

The union of crowns to fill a void of a missing tooth or teeth

This is almost an element of the past because of implants.

If the teeth surrounding the missing tooth are in need of restoration, a bridge will provide a union of crowns but requires different types of home care. Remember, man-made products just do not quite hold up as well as the real stuff, and require special care. Floss needs to go under the free hanging crown. Just think of a road and bridge structure. Support is on two sides and built up and designed to hold a force in the middle by not giving way to weight being applied in the middle.

Any time the body finds something in or near it that it does not like, it will try to package it up and push it to the outside world for ejection. Think of a thorn. When the bridge structure is made in the lab, the tissue in the middle where the tooth WAS is used to support the pressure on the Pontic. The Pontic is the free standing crown in the middle that fills in the missing tooth. When food is left under the Pontic, the body will react by pulling away from either a natural or man made area of infection. This will allow the bridge to bend slightly during chewing. The teeth on either side are pushed and pulled in directions they were not designed to go. The natural teeth under the crowns on the sides of the bridge; that are only trying to help, will be waddled right out of their slots.

Think of it this way. If you went to get the mail everyday, and you took hold of the mail box and gave it a good shake, then day after day, after week, that mailbox would have a hard time standing there no matter the underlining support. Treat your teeth like that and they will Bend-Crack-Break or just hurt during usage. Teeth are designed only for slight movement side to side or up and down. Stressful movement will cause trouble; bridges do break off teeth that were used for support. No welding can be done in the mouth. So, if things go bad and cracks or decay damages the support to your bridge, there goes your expensive investment! All of the structure comes out an all new items have to be purchased.

BRIDGE THREADERS are available almost everywhere. With the old style you have to add the string floss to it yourself (like threading a needle for some of us). Or you can buy them ready-built that cost a little more but are still CHEAPER THAN DENTAL APPOINTMENTS. Your mother always told you to take care of the things you have.

Root Canals:

Removal of the diseased nerve from the canal within which the nerve lives and the bacteria that has taken up residence

As the nerve supply leaves the spine (lets call it the trunk of a tree), it will branch out to supply most of the area from the ear to the lips. Not too surprising to hear, a patient will refer to discomfort a little off from the area of the infection. Patient will point to the top tooth when asked where it hurts. X-rays will show no problem in that area, but the presence of an infection will be visible on the bottom jaw.

Bacteria enter the mouth with every breath in search of a home and food. The filmy, sticky surface on the tooth is room and board. Any thing that eats will have waste; this waste is very acidic and will melt the tooth. The hole in the tooth is of no interest to the bacteria other than providing a larger table for which to find the next meal, until the size of the hole reaches the blood and nerve supply. This is the canal formed by the body to protect and nurture the tooth. Bacteria think it has been invited to the banquet of a lifetime, and the limitations are only within the boundaries of the entire blood supply. That means head to toe. First, the bacteria will have the ability to get rid of its waste, by your swallowing, but when the cavity has been plugged by food, or anything; an opened into the jaw bone will be created by the acidy of the pus. Pressure builds as the waste builds and there is no room for the bacteria, blood, waste, and the body's defense system. The nerve endings are pushed up against the bone, or squeezed by the pus. Nerve get mad and tell the brain "I have had enough, get something done." Brain decides it needs outside help and will continue to send out messages of distress till assistance is provided. Pain will keep you up, make your body hurt and maybe this is why you can't get your blood sugar to stabilize. Or your joints could hurt a little more intensely. If the infection really gets a foothold on the bodies defenses, the side of the face can swell up within hours to where there seems to be no neck. Get ready; the bacteria will go for the main supply of food, the heart, or the brain, where there is unknown results. None of the possibilities are listed on the vacation brochures.

Medical Emergency can only assist in temporary relief.
(Drugs will only kill off the nerd version of the bacteria.)
(Eating and breathing will feed the reason for the pain.)

A Dentist can provide the only long term positive results.
The tooth will heal with the medication that is left by the dentist. Teeth will also dry out because the blood supply has been terminated, therefore leaving the tooth drier and increasing the chance to break. It is not just the body's bones that will break as we age, teeth will also break.

Apicoectomy:

Surgery to remove the root tip

A small window is open on the cheek side below the tooth exposing the root of the tooth and the area of the infection. A section of bone and the root tip is removed in hopes of saving the tooth. A root canal is generally preformed before this is attempted, because it is less invasive and less facial structure is involved. Since implants, this has become less frequent because of expense, and because the chance of failure is still possible. It is commonly used when removing a defect or tumor, caused by trauma, such as an impact to the tooth's support. (Tumors can appear many, many years after an impact trauma occurs to a boney region.) Caution needs to be taken in the area of the lower jaw's nerve, numbness might be permanent. There is no guarantee that this will stop the pain, it is expensive, and the money might best be invested in an **implant** on a root canalled tooth. I can tell you that I have had an Apico on a front tooth, with success.

Extraction

"Just pull the thing; I have others I can use to eat a meal."

The teeth fit into the jaw like interlacing the extended fingers on the right hand in the extended fingers of the left hand. Two boney surfaces just don't live in harmony when movement is involved. Think of two pieces of chalk that are rubbed together. To prevent the destruction of the tooth or the jaw, the body has designed a shock absorber to provide a cushion. Just as everywhere else in the body, such as, a ligament in elbow/knees. How many of us have not injured one of these areas, and limped or babied the area for days?   The Periodontal Ligament (Perio means mouth) is the shock absorber that grabs hold of the jaw on one side and the tooth on the other. You have felt this body part talking every time you have something stuck between your teeth, though it might only be as thick as a hair, it will feel like a telephone pole to your brain.

To remove a tooth the dentist must release these attachments (ligaments) slowly to save as much of the jaw bone in its place as possible. The removal of every tooth will reduce the fullness of the face, and increase wrinkles. YES, the loss of a tooth will create a void. This void will be healed by the natural functions of the body, a boney scab. The area where the tooth was will be filled with blood and an element that will act like logs in a running river. Platelets in the blood will instantly start creating a very soft mushy scab, filling the entire W or U shape area, with healing elements. If the healing is not disturbed and allowed to perform as the body has intended, you can return to most of your daily routine. Rinse the area with warm salty water the **NEXT** day. Brush the area very gently with a **soft** tooth brush about three days after extraction and be careful with sharp food, like chips.

Follow instructions:

Do not **smoke** (if you have to, just take a couple of short puffs)

Do not **spit**

Do not use a **straw.**

All of these actions create suction in the mouth and pull at the scab.

These three item are important for 12 hrs

Don't drink soda's for 3 days (breaks down the scalp)

Please don't eat anything that is too **small** (falls in the hole) or too **hot** (dissolves the scab).

> If the bleeding is too much, just place a
> WARM tea bag over the extraction site.

Dry Sockets:
If the scab is disturbed after the tooth is removed.

The body has put forth a lot of effort to create this scab; it will not do it again. Next it will lay down a thin scab that will use the design of the bone to hold it in place. Remember the interlacing fingers, pull away the right hand and view the spaces the left hands fingers; the new scab will follow this shape in a thin line. The socket where the tooth lived was always moist, now it is dry. That's right, a DRY SOCKET. The nice soft scab would have taken a couple of days for the tenderness to subside. In a dry socket it will take the body about three months to fill the area, building layer after layer, slowly filling up the void. The discomfort of a dry socket will show up on the third or fourth day. The pain will be equal to a very bad toothache. Raw bone is exposed to all the PH and temperatures of the mouth. Yes, food will fall into the void and create a very bad odor.

If someone says: "I just could not stand the taste of that blood in my mouth, I had to spit!" What did you do the last time you cut your finger? Place the bloody finger in your mouth, did you? Blood is blood it will all taste the same; it comes from the same heart! Just how clean was your finger when you cut it? Three months will be needed for healing a DRY SOCKET.

After Extractions
  Go home
  Get in the recliner.
  It is good to keep the head higher than the heart
  Sleep
  Take the medication if it was provided by the doctor

Grab the remote and eat plain ice cream
  (remember the not to small pieces)

DRY SOCKETS NEED TO BE SEEN BY THE DENTIST
SO CHEMICALS CAN BE PLACED IN THE SOCKET
TO INCREASE MOISTURE AND HEALING

Space Maintainers

Fixed Unilateral: One or more teeth are missing, to hold the space a loop of wire is used like a kickstand (one side of face)

Fixed Bilateral: To hold space on both sides of the top OR bottom jaw where many teeth are missing

Recement of space maintainer: this is a man made device Placed on with a man make chemical There are just foods that will pop the glue loose.

When baby (pedo) teeth are lost early because of decay, abscess or accident, the space where the tooth was, needs to be held for the adult tooth. Think of it as a parking lot with pre-set strips during holiday shopping. Organization is more likely to be controlled with designated parking of the cars.

Could you just imagine how the parking lot would look if you could just pull up, get out, and hoping that there would be room to back out when you return?

It's the same with adult teeth. As the facial plates grow and the width of the adult teeth is twice that of the baby teeth, guidance is needed.

Baby teeth hold the space so that the neighboring teeth will not drift over into areas that they just were not meant to occur. The top teeth hammer on the bottom and vice/versa, encouraging drift and movement.

Front adult teeth are visible at birth in an x-ray. The buds are starting to form.

If you could just look at the x-ray of a preschool child, you could see not only the teeth that they are using, but all the teeth that will be in the future. It looks like a stack of rock piled up in the garden. (20 baby/ 28 adult, plus maybe wisdom teeth)

Please just watch the diet at all ages. Keeping your own teeth is one of the star players in growing old with grace. Years ago, an eighty nine year old lady came toddling in with her granddaughter. She was wearing one of those smiles that just made you want to hug her, and join in on the happiness of life.

She looked up at me "You know I am not afraid of dying. Know Why?

When I get to heaven; Gods going to give me back my teeth; so I can really eat a meal again."

Dentures are like eating a meal where the biting surface is either sloshing around or pinching on the soft pink tissue. Just try in those teeth that can be picked up during Halloween. You will get the gist of it.

**CARE FOR YOUR CHILDRENS TEETH
THEY ARE IMPORTANT
BE GENTLE AND THOROUGH**

Dentures (Partials Are Just Part Of A Denture)

ARE YOU A HAPPY HIKER WHEN YOUR RIGHT SHOE IS TWO SIZES TO BIG AND THE LEFT SHOE TWO SIZES TO SMALL? Dentures will either pinch or slouch around with every bite. This will become every more obvious as the day of use increase. Taste buds are all over the mouth. Cover them up with any kind of object and you will lose much of the flavor you have been accustomed too.

Sure they will be the color of teeth you have always dreamed of and will be straight and evenly sized. Easy to use? Well, have you ever tried to eat a meal on a roller skate? The lower jaw oscillates on a hinge, the most solicited joint in the entire body. The upper plate will stay in with suction, but consider the items that will get under the plate and feel like a thorn: anything with a small seed, tomatoes, berries.

"Well I just eat sandwiches anyway," you may say. I hope you like old bread! The new soft textured bread will stick to the top of your mouth and stay there until you pull out the plate and pry the white paste off. You will be familiar with the location of every public restroom. Maybe you can use the grandchild as an excuse.

But you never have to worry about pizza burn again; the roof of your mouth is now covered with hard plastic. Your toughest meat will be in meatloaf form, and for the raw vegetables that are good for digestion, you need to buy a blender.

Some have said "I eat anything I want."

No You Swallow Anything You Want.

Next is upper and lower GI Problems.

A dentist said "Wish I could charge double for the top and give the lower teeth for free. When the patients say they hate the bottom teeth, I could just say."

"Well they were free."

Most lower dentures are kept in pockets and bathroom drawers. As one person put it, "I wear them to church and for family pictures."

Dentures fit onto the jawbone like a saddle goes on a horse. There has to be a thick enough horse to hold the saddle. The earlier in life one goes into a denture, the less likely there will be a strong enough horse to put a saddle on later in life. The facial bone is a trabecular bone which means it has air holes. Our skinny little neck would not be able to hold up our cannonball size head any other way. This type of bone has a honeycomb structure. Wearing a denture hits directly on this surface to provide the chewing pressure, and the honeycomb cavities are crushed over time.

Eventually, your **nose** and your **chin** become best friends.

If you do not wait too long, implants can be considered, provided there is enough bone to place them into. Implants need support and enough bone for the fixture to infiltrate, thereby stabilizing the titanium substance to the jaw, discussed later in implant section

Two Types of Dentures

First: Immediate Denture
                 Teeth are pulled and denture is placed immediately
                 Dentures have been prepared by the information
                 collected in the past visits
Advantages: Dentures act as a bandage over extraction site
                 Always have a smile
                 Always have something to assist chewing
Disadvantages: Hard Plastic placed on top of stitches,
                 immediately
                 Healing of the extraction site and
                 becoming accustomed to dentures together
                 Food trapped under dentures and irritating healing
                 Needs relined after healing a couple
                 of months: extra cost, maybe

Second: Extraction site is allowed to heal 4 to 6 months before denture delivered
                 Advantages: Sure fit
                 First stage is healing and discomfort over
                 Reline needed 3 to 5 years
                 Disadvantages: Months without chewing assistants
                 Jaw placement is off and could cause facial muscles stress

Valplast upgrade: The metal frame work with pink tips that reaching out and hold on to the natural tooth, keeping the partial in position. Or, all of the plastic will be upgraded to the softer product. Real plus is when the partial starts moving around; you simply place in a warm bowl of water for a couple of minutes, and then allow cooling in your mouth; snug fit again with no trip to the dental office. There is an addition expense to the metal denture cost.

All dentures need relining if there is weight change of (plus/minus) 10 pounds.

Every 3 to 5 years liner against the tissue needs to be refreshed.

Every 5 to 10 years the plastic teeth need to be replaced

That's right, plastic teeth wear out fast

So you could chose porcelain, they last longer.

Porcelain teeth will sound like two teacups clicking together.

Try this clicking sound out, before requesting this sound in your daily talking.

Partial means part of a denture. Step for producing and care are much the same.

Roof of the mouth will be covered with metal or plastic. The lower teeth will have something around the tongue, to balance out the rocking motion produced when biting on one side. There are single tooth partials that do work well, but need just as much care.

Snap- On Smile

Seen any of the movies or shows that have the vampires? Their added extent on to the eye teeth can be product quickly with this cosmetics product. Think of the Halloween teeth that have been around for decades, but use the beauty and craftsmanship of today's dental labs. People that work in dental labs are trained just like the craftsmen's of fine jewelry. This finished product will snap over your existing teeth, therefore add thickness to the over-all face, and will drive your tongue crazy for a couple of weeks. Excellent product to consider if you are in the process of implants healing, rampant decay from maybe cancer therapy and need to keep up that beautiful smile in public. Cost is in the thousands. Home care must be very pin point quality, to assure the longevity of the good teeth being use for the snap-on function.

Again**, HOME CARE Must Be Very GOOD.** This is not a denture. It is a quick fix to replace an open space or spaces. People thinking that a full mouth of crowns, twenty years ago, was the way to produce that picture perfect smile, falsely believed this would be their last investment. Some who were not taught or did not follow the direction provide, found that huge investment crashed into an expensive unhappiness.

The life span of a crown is only twenty years by design. When things start failing it can be like a snowball in an avalanche, watching one tooth crash; one after another. This is the perfect situation for a Snap- on smile. The overall product is a single unit. As the teeth fail and or become weak, the unity of all the teeth will be crutched together, can sometimes is beneficial.

Just like anything else in the medical, patient are the test tubes of our education and will always be the providers of side effects and reason for continually changing and improving products and changing education.

Patients have told me, after some of the explanations of their situation,

"I think I will just go back and sue that Dentist"

You can not sue someone that was providing STANDARD OF CARE for that day in time; by the education we are able to provide today.

Even in the show Star Trek. "Can you believe those barbarians cut people open and did savage surgery?" Maybe in the year 2525 we will just walk into a closet and have dental surgery done by light beams that will reconstruct our broken parts.

Implants:

MANKIND'S STEP FOR SAVING THE T-BONE STEAK DIET

You may have wanted to hang pictures on the part of the wall where there is no stud board under the sheetrock to support the weight of the frame. There is a small devise that can be inserted; sometimes it takes a couple of them to provide the support to make the frame stable. This same design is used to attach an implant to the jaw bone.

This is the way I try to describe the placement of implants to the patient.

Step: Picture Hanger	Implant Part
1. Plastic is placed into the sheetrock	Titanium implant
2. Long screw is tightened in plastic part	Abutment
3. Desired decoration is hung on the wall	Crown

The titanium implant is placed with care by the doctor at just the right angle to work in conjunction with all bone, teeth and tissue in the surrounding area. Healing cap in placed over the insert and the body is allowed to continue in its normal healing process. Later the union between the implant and the crown will be inserted: the abutment. The crown is attached to the abutment. How the teeth come together is checked.

Off you go to enjoy a T-bone steak dinner. Immediate load of the crown, to the implant can be discussed, with the doctor, in some cases.

Implants can return you to the smile you had in high school, or the one you wished you had. An enhanced chewing ability is also part of the bonus package. Without implants, when teeth are lost, the sharp point of every corn chip will attack the soft, delicate tissue left behind in the open spaces. You really discover the true strength and ability of the jaw and teeth when teeth are missing and the pink stuff starts taking on the texture of the food.

An individual implant will fill the void and provide the function of a lost tooth, but it must be kept out of the direct force that the overall jaw creates because of its structural design. It is manmade so not as flexible as a real tooth. The overall force of a bite must be distributed. This is the reason for mutable implants placement in dentures.

With full arch implants-four/eight to an arch-the load-bearing pressure is spread over a greater distance and their stability is greatly improved. There is almost the same ability as natural chewing. Limitations occur when time has passed, and the thickness of the jaw is not deep enough to insert an implant. The new mini implant does not require too much bone, but the nail can not be longer than the board. With mini-implants more are needed. The cost per unit is less but the increase in numbers makes the cost sometimes the same.

The cost of implants for a full mouth is about the same as a new car and almost the cost of a house, depending on just how fancy you want to get. No monthly payment will be accepted at almost any dental office. WHY? Because you walk out with the total product, and repossession is unheard of.

(Recently, a credit card company came up with an installment plan with no interest, IF you pay back in a limited amount of months.)

THE COST IS HIGH BUT YOU WILL BE USING IMPLANTS FOR EATING DAILY. There are cheaper ways to eat a meal, but this type of replacement will provide the beauty and chewing ability you had as a teenager or always dreamed of. As one patient put it, "It's got to feel better than what the stock market is doing to me."

THORTON FLOSSERS are available and are the best product for cleaning and maintaining the health of your implant, in my opinion. They did not pay me to say that. Maybe they should. The ones in the pink box are designed for implants and work great on bridges.

They are a little pricey but just how much did you pay for that implant; take care of it.

This is a book about common sense dentistry

General Knowledge That's Good To Know

START EARLY IN TEACHING HOW TO CARE FOR TEETH

DON'T JUST TALK, SET AN EXAMPLE

YOUR TEETH MIGHT BE HOPELESS BUT
CARE FOR WHAT YOU HAVE

KIDS WILL COPY WHAT IS SEEN WITHOUT
YOU SAYING A WORD

Baby Teeth

Message the gums even before teeth appear in the mouth. This will get the child accustom to having something in his or her mouth, it will clean the soft baby food off the gums; and it will make your life easier in the future with tooth brushing.

Start cleaning your baby's teeth after a meal, while he or she is still in the high chair. This is also great for teething. Just let them chew on the brush while in the chair. Let the child brush first, and then follow up with an adult brushing the teeth, gently on all sides. Help your children to brush their teeth until sometime in their third year of school.

Floss your child's teeth

If there is one thing that will keep your teeth
health for life: it is flossing.
As soon as there are two teeth, floss the space between them.

When children sit down for their, lets say, favorite TV show, have them floss or brush and develop a habit. Ask them to message the teeth and gum or remove the thing between their teeth. You want something (health smile); they want their favorite down time.

Fluoride should be use the first night a tooth is seen in the mouth. Fluoride only works when it can touch a **clean** tooth surface. ACT, a children fluoride rinse, can be applied with a Q-tip on clean teeth at bedtime, before the child learns to rinse and spit. This is a big added bonus for a health smile in the future. I understand the concerns with chemical and children. But, there is so much benefit to having good teeth, and with today's snack choices; teeth need extensive help. Parents might be handing out all the best of snack choices, but children loves sweets and they will except treats from many other people. There is no other chemical that can fortify a tooth more than Fluoride, day to day.

Why care for the short lived 'Baby Teeth'?

Some people may say, "Well, they are going to lose the baby teeth. Why do I have to care for them?" For one reason, you help your children avoid losing sleep from the pain of cavities. One important job of the baby teeth, besides eating, is to hold space in the mouth for the proper placement of adult teeth. Think of a parking lot with no stripes for the Christmas shoppers. Many cars end up parked in a way that is a disadvantages to others who wish to park. Teeth, if left on their own without the support of prearranged parking, are likely to drift into any open spaces. If you want to assure the need for braces, just avoid caring for and repairing the baby teeth as needed. Baby teeth taken out because of problems will lose the guide path for the future permanent teeth.

True, it's a boring job; you are working backward with limited vision. But it pays long term dividends for your child.

Finish all bottles in an upright position and clean the mouth afterwards. Yes, even before teeth appear in the mouth. Children have the habit of falling asleep with the content still pooled in the cheek and tongue area. The sweeteners, even if natural, will not do the teeth any good.

When should my child have teeth?

Timing on when children's teeth showing up will vary. There are some patterns that are set up, but don't worry about when teeth appear. Have more concerns on keeping the mouth clean from the first day food is placed in the infant's mouth.

Chemicals used for teething

Please review the information recently provided by the FDA. Strong warning have be posted against such compounds.

Teresa Kay

Child's Visit To A Dentist

The child's first visit to a dental office could just be a ride in the chair, getting to touch different tooth brush types, and happily visiting with the dental team and getting used to the experience.

A dental hygienist might brush the child's teeth and floss and even apply a protective varnish (this component can be swallowed with no problem). The child's should be seen by a dentist after their **second birthday**, or **anytime** you have a concerns.

Be aware that the dentist and technicians will work close to the child's face, Take that into consideration when you make an appointment and try to make all positive comparisons with each step that will be provided when talking to the child.

The second visit to the dentist could be a full visit, with a polishing of the teeth, flossing and a visual view of teeth by the dentist. X-rays are uncomfortable at all ages, so that, too, should be taken under consideration. It is very important to use X-rays in setting up a treatment plan. It is also important for parents to develop a comfortable relationship with your dental team, so the child can see your friendship and confidence.

A third visit to the dentist could provide the opportunity for the dentist to develop a full set of records. Please try to let the child have a few happy visits before a restorative visit is needed. It will help the child develop a stronger lifelong stability with his or her teeth.

Many medications can be provided to children to help them have a relaxing visit with the dentist during fillings. Your dentist has the license of DDS- Doctor of Dental Surgery. Work done to the teeth **is surgery**, just preformed under local anesthesia. Remember that with good home care and early happy visits, it is possible that only nitrous oxide gas be used for restorative visits. If there is a lot of work to be done, or if the child will not sit in the chair with limited movement, other options are available for calming or restraint. This is so the dental staff can <u>HELP</u> the child return to comfortable eating ability. When children are not seen by the dental team in a timely manner, the first visit can lead to a lot of work that needs to be completed. Hospital admission with full sedation is also an option for moderate to severe cases. This procedure will be preformed by a dentist with an added degree and licenses that allows him to work in the hospital. Now it is easy to understand the surgery part but the only difference is the amount of work done within the time limits, and the number of chemical used to provide comfort.

One child told me that their teeth hurt all the time, made them cry and loose sleep.   **But one day I woke up and I had all this jewelry in my mouth and No Pain.**

Everyone will be in a dental office sooner or later, except those who only postpone the event by being in the garage with pliers with the hope of not fainting, or those at the liquor store asking, "Which brand works best for toothaches?" That root tip, the broken off part left in the jaw, will need to be taken out by a dentist.

Please help your children remove loose teeth. As the tooth lifts, food can become trapped under and creates an environment that is undesirable to the new tooth. Yes, new adult teeth can be born with first stages of decay.

PLEASE NEVER USE DENTAL VISITS AS A WEAPON IN
TEACHING CHILDREN ANYTHING
THE DENTIST IS THE ONLY HOPE IN REDUCING DENTAL
PAIN

Never Use The Word Shot

Positive comments:
    The doctor will put the tooth to sleep
      Just like when you sit on your foot to long
    When the tooth is asleep
      The doctor will place a band-aid over the hurt tooth

Behavioral Management:
Tooth structures are a very hard material. Teeth have to be to handle all the items that are placed in there for nutrition and habits. When repair is needed the instruments will be sharp, moving at a very high speed, and soft tissue can be harmed. Keeping still so that the procedure can be completed quickly, efficiently and safely is critical. If extra hands, personnel or articles are needed there might be a charge. Quite often there is a referral to specialist. Repair of a very sick tooth could save your child life and improve their health

Anesthesia:
Dentistry is a better world with chemistry. In very few events in life does someone get in your face, place their hands all over you and leave you numb.

With the introduction of the breathable gas nitrous, a patient can be placed in a semi-conscious state and leave with little side effect. Just make sure you are left on pure oxygen for ten minutes and allowed to set up and or stand up without being dizzy.

N2O: (Nitrous oxide) Breathable gas that will provide a feeling of light sleep. It is charge by the minute or hours. This is not a cheap drug. The person that is sitting in the room must have a license to even be there when the doctor has stepped out.

Oral Habits

These include thumb, fingers, pacifier or any other object that is placed in the mouth. I believe it is necessary to wait and use positive reinforcement and reasoning, during the years in kindergarten. Suggest the teacher join in on the progress in remind the child to avoid the oral habit and provide the treat (new class puzzle).

Allow the child to pick out a Grand Prize. Place a picture of the object on a board with 30-40 boxes below. Each time the habit is seen during the day, ask the child to hold or stand by the picture. At night, place something to cover the thumb and fingers so the child will be aware of the habit, and try to stop; place blanket or pacifier near by, but not taken away. In the morning if the habit is avoided, make a big deal of placing a sticker one of the boxes.

A habit can be developed or broken in 30 days. It will help if there is small prizes every 5-7 stickers, that the family can participate in; ice cream, movies, or pizza. If there is no success within wait a couple of weeks and try again in a couple of months, or bring the prize into the house, insight but out of reach. Each child develops reasoning at a different pace. Try to stay positive.

KIDS GRINDING TEETH

Parents, this question come up often; it's just a phase that some kids go through. I think they are working the adult teeth into the needed position. Hopefully, most kids will stop when all adult teeth are in position**. It is when this habit continues into the adult teeth that concerns arise.** Treatment for a child might interfere with the natural facial growth of a developing child facial shape.

Stains

Here are a few reasons for different stains and just how to remove them.

Coffee and Tea stains are the easiest to remove but must be done regularly. This stain is very superficial (on top of tooth) and can be removed with the uses of baking soda. Yes, just the kind that is used about the house for cooking, cleaning and keeping things fresh. Brush with baking soda a couple of times a week before using your toothpaste. The toothpaste with baking soda just does not have enough to remove some of the stubborn stain of the heavier tea and coffee drinkers. Hot tea and instant coffee will stain more that the other products. If it has been to long and the stain has become a little stubborn, add hydrogen peroxide to a little baking soda in the palm of your hand, and brush your teeth. This mixture must be fresh.

All foods or drinks that have a color can stain the teeth. This includes carrots, spinach and any other products that are rich in color. Darker colored vegetables are better for our diet and need to be consumed daily. Baking soda will remove these stains if used a couple of times a week.

Black line stain is a by product of consuming a health bit of iron. Iron is an essential mineral in the production of red blood cells. Iron is found in strawberries, spinach, dark green vegetables and organ meats. Some individuals need to increase this element in their diet to maintain a health state or just like to eat these health products. The stain will appear in the lower front teeth and cheek side of the top back teeth. A baking soda with hydrogen peroxide mixture used a couple of times a week, will reduce the staining. Complete removal will require a professional cleaning in a dental office.

Yellow or Orange stain along the area where the tooth meets the gum, is seen frequently.   This is caused by not brushing the teeth for a couple of week. Green will appear when it has been a month of more, since the last brushing.

This one is easy to prevent. BRUSH DAILY.

Tobacco stain is an aromatic stain. This stain will pierce deep into the structure of the tooth. To remove this stain the products for bleaching teeth will need to be purchased. (See section on bleaching.)

Tobacco Products

No, this is not a section that will scold you for your habit. If you have not heard it is bad you, you have not been of this generation or maybe this planet. I will ask you to use a little common sense and check your tissue regularly.

First, if you are a smoker, try not to take such long, hard drags on the cigarette. The heat created from the flame will cook the inside of the mouth. Just like placing a piece of meat in the pan and flipping it over quickly. This tissue is traumatized and will not inform you, as quickly, if something is going wrong in the mouth. This is why you might not know that the gums are bleeding from gum disease, because the tissue is cauterized.

Tobacco products will produce a type of chemical reaction to the tissue. The tissue will set off its early warning system, if you are lucky. Take the finger and insert them into the corner of the lips. Bite down and take a good look at the tissue between the cheek and the teeth. (Review the section on oral cancer exam.) If you see a white, lacey area, looks like cottage cheese, maybe. When you touch it, it will move and stick to your finger. This could be cancer, stage one. Please have the area checked as soon as possible, by a medical professional. Stop all tobacco products; or at least cut way back. It is wise not place the tobacco product in the same spot every time; move it around. This includes the spot where the cigarette rest on the lips.

Staining on the teeth will come from the heat and the air picking up the tobacco color. Professional grade products will need to be provided by a dental office, to have the white teeth, you are hoping to achieve.

A Gap In My Front Teeth

Do you have a space between the front two teeth on the top? The separation of these teeth is caused by a very strong muscle. Lift the upper lip; look at the area between the soft tissue of the lip and the boney structure that holds the teeth, in this area a thin line of tissue extending out, in a semi-circle which attaches to both types of tissue. Everyone has these muscles; they are located in several spots around the upper and lower jaw area. Sometimes this muscle is very thick; it can extend deep into the boney structure holding the teeth, causing them to have a gap. This strong muscle does have the possibilities to be passed from generation to generation. An Oral Surgeon can simple clip the tissue early in a child developmental years and reduce the width of the gap. (Fernectomy)

The frentom is this muscles name. There are other problems this muscle can cause, just in front of the tooth where this muscle is position. Recession is the loss of tissue that covers the front of the tooth. This muscle could pull and tug at this tissue on the tooth and cause a loss of coverage on the tooth. The teeth resist the pressure applied by the tongue, with every swallow, by the strength of the muscle in the lip and the strength of the thin muscle covering the front of the teeth. Lose one and the pressure of the tongue has to ability to push the teeth forward.

Tongue tied is the most common reason for this procedure. The slim layer of tissue under the tongue has developed in a way that restricts the movement of the tongue. The tongue should be able to touch the roof of the mouth when the mouth is open wide. Is also should be able to be extended out pass the lips. Restriction of the tongue will cause speech and chewing limitation. Surgery will involve numbing the area and cutting the flap of tissue, which has simple over developed.

How We Chew!

The tongues job is to push food outward to the teeth. Cheeks and lips job is to push food inward toward the tongue. Jaw mashes the food. The saliva moisturizes the mouth to make swallowing easier, enzymes in the saliva also starts the digestive process. When the tongue and throat feel like the particles of food are small enough to prevent gagging; swallowing is allowed.

When teeth are lost the tongue needs to swell out to the cheek region to assist in the movement of food. The tongue will also learn to maneuver food in the region of remaining teeth. Missing teeth might be the reason you bite your tongue more.

Back teeth are designed to be the work horses. They are wider and have more legs to stand on. (Top teeth 3 roots, lower teeth 2 roots) Front teeth only have one skinny leg (root). They are designed for cutting through and tearing. Force the front teeth to do the load of a work horse and they will become loose over time.

It is like going for the mail and giving the mailbox a good shake before walking off. It does not matter the type of support, sooner or latter, things will start to fall.

Orthodontic: Braces

Teeth fit into the jaw like interlacing fingers. The two boney materials will not work without the spacing between them, or they will rub each other to oblivion. This space is filled with a shock absorber that grabs hold of the jawbone and the tooth and pulls them together. When a tooth needs to be moved to a position that looks attractive to you, and is in good functional position for the dental structure, these ligaments will be the key factor. The body has the ability to build and destroy bone by using elements called osteocytes and osteoblasts. A bracket for the movement of the tooth is put in place, so that this point of the tooth will eventually be in the desired position. Wires push and pull the tooth into the desired position; light wires are used at first. Slow and Steady.

Monthly dental visits are needed to increase the strength of the wire and replace the small rubber bands that hold the wire into the bracket. Here you thought the cute little colors that were associated with braces were part of the child motivation process. Inside the jaw the periodontal ligaments are being pulled on one side of the tooth and smashed on the opposite side. At first the jaw will just complain about the discomfort and ask the body to consider a change. When no change is resolved in a day or so, the bone in the mouth will start changing to resolve the discomfort. On the side with pressure, the bone will dissolve; the side with the strain will start building bone. Just about the time the jaw has fixed all the discomfort, it is time for another dental visit.

At some point the teeth will need to be placed in harmony with the opposing jaw. Rubber bands will be placed on hooks from top to bottom in triangle or box positions. Yes these bands break and go flying. I asked my kids not to look straight at me when talking to me during this time of their braces. They said, "Mom, you should feel what it is like to have them fire off in your mouth." If the patient does not wear the rubber bands as instructed, this phase of the procedure is never achieved. To help the person understand why this is important, make comparisons. One comparison is the video games. You are trying to get to the next level, but you just didn't choose the right door. The game is over and you must start back at the previous level.

Some teeth will refuse to be born and lock in position deep in the jaw. This will require surgery to open a window, place a bracket on the top of the buried tooth and use a tow chain to pull it to position during braces. **All for the sake of beauty?** All tissue in the body has its place. When in disarray, sometime undesirable events occur. Nothing listed on a vacation brochure.

"It seems like the teeth are straight. Why won't the doctor take them off?"

It will take a little time for the bone to ensure placement of the tooth. Very good home care will decrease the time in braces and increase the stability of the repositioned tooth. When the surrounding tissue of the tooth is sick with gum disease the tooth might think, "Well I was not sick in the old position, let's drift back!" Therefore, the reason for a retainer, kids will be kids.

Retainers:

A devise to keep teeth in that position
That means held, not moved

These are devices that hold the positions for teeth that exist at that moment and time. If you like the way teeth look after braces, wear your retainer. No marry your retainer! At least wear it a couple of nights a week. If you leave it out for a couple of days and it hurts to wear it, this means the teeth are drifting back to their original position. They will never forget where they were born. Let gum disease develop late in life and the teeth will still remember where they were born.

"Maybe, there is no sick tissue where we were!"

Once a month someone comes in and asks,

"Can just this one tooth can be pushed back?"

My question: "What put it in that position?"

Patient: "Braces"

My reply: "That's what it will take to open the parking space for that tooth."

WEAR YOUR RETAINER, MARRY YOUR RETAINER

NEVER PLACE IT IN A PAPER PRODUCT.

Place it your shirt, bra or somewhere it will bother you after the meal.

Put it back in your mouth where it belongs.(if your are wearing it during the day)

It could get accidentally thrown away.

I suggest applying moisturing mouth spray with enzymes, added protection. Taste is better in the morning. Sprinkle with baking soda during storage.

Wisdom Teeth

I have seen x-rays where a wisdom tooth is on its side, sticking out toward the cheek, or headed toward the ear. I saw a teenage when I was still in college who had eight wisdom teeth, stacked, one atop the other. The surgeon had to take out the first four, and then let the jaw heal for a couple of years. The removal of the second set was to take place when they were in late twenties.

Now, if any of you have had wisdom teeth taken out, one of the big pluses is that it will never be an event that you have to experience again. Not this one!

Extraction of wisdom teeth is best done at a young age, just when the top (crown) of the tooth is completely formed and the legs (roots) start to form, and all of this is under the gums. The dentist will be able to detect if there is enough room for the addition of another tooth. This tooth must have enough room to <u>fully erupt</u> into the mouth and be reached for daily home care. The bone is a lot more pliable at a younger age and the harder cortical bone has not formed around the root. If you look at a younger person's x-ray, you can see the saddle separating the legs of the tooth starting to form. Removal of wisdom teeth at this time is called the sweet spot for extractions. Less resistance, they seem to roll out easier, and healing is easier and faster at this younger age.

I once took an 85 year old to emergency for a mild stroke the evening after a wisdom tooth was removed. "Well it is only a tooth," some might say. "Well, it's only a finger. You have others. It's no big deal to cut one of them off, is it?"

The teeth are only how far from the brain
WHICH REGISTERS EVERYTHING

When teeth hurt from infection, just remember, you are allowing pus to grow freely into an area with small openings like a honeycomb. This infection does have a class system, from nerd to superman version. IF the more powerful superman version has the best luck in reproducing, that's when your face will swell up like a horror movie, special effects monster. A hospital emergency is not set up to pull teeth. Coming to the dentist with a swollen face, is little help either. Swelling is thick with components similar to lard and acid. The chemical to make it numb is like water. You can't push water into lard and make a nerve go to sleep. So you just have to wait till the swelling goes down. Good luck sleeping.

Home Care For Dentures And Partials

More needs to be done, that just placing the denture in the nightly soaking compound. (Check for ADA symbol) This tissue in the mouth was accustom to fresh air moving over the area, regularly. Now the tissue in trapped under a hard plastic, which can collect, food and bacteria. There are bacteria that live in the mouth and are considered healthy, flora. Flora can contain as many as 700 different types of organisms. Flora is a well managed organism that is a balance of all the good and bad guys. When one or another is allowed to develop and thrive, could this lead to other health problems? Makes sense to me! Under the plastic, an environment is created that will allow certain one to thrive. This will be evident if the tissue under the denture is red, slick and puffy. To stabilize the tissue, removal of the denture once or twice a week for over night, would be helpful. There are those that just can not sleep without the denture, or will not be seen without a denture in place. This is okay.

Yogurt has all the good guys and in a perfect balance for the oral tissue. This is one time you will be ask to play with your food. After the nightly home care regiment of brushing, flossing and cleaning the denture, brush the gum part of your mouth, where the teeth are missing and with the denture or partial out of your mouth; slowly eat yogurt. With each bite allow the organism in the yogurt to come in contact with the tissue for a short period of time.

In nightly home care, here is where a hard toothbrush is needed, but not in the mouth. There are custom made brushes for dentures. They are double ended; flat side with hard bristles for the plastic teeth, and an area with pointed bristles for the side that will rest against the tissue. A good dishwashing detergent is good for the over all denture. Rinse well.

Partials are simple part of a denture.

Care must be provided to the metal or plastic clasp (Valplast) around the teeth. The innocent teeth, under the claps, are now asked to do the work of the missing teeth. Extra pressure is place on them, in a direction; they were not built to receive.

Extra food will now be collecting around the clap, because they do not conform to the design of natural teeth. A <u>small child toothbrush</u> needs to be used in the areas of the missing teeth, to message the tissue and brush the **all sides** of the exposed teeth. Then coat the sides of the teeth with <u>Fluoride every night on the surface of a clean tooth.</u>

Facial Bone Structure And Toothaches

If you had a balloon and pencils poking into the balloon very gently, you could envision how the sinuses and the tooth roots live in harmony.

The root of the tooth has a nerve and a blood supply all squeezing in boney membranes between the sinuses and the tip of the tooth. When the sinuses are clean, and nothing is draining down your throat or being blown out your nose, there is a normal flow of nutrients and signals between the body and the tooth. When the allergy season, or colds and flu arrive and fill the air you're breathing with pollen, viruses, or bacteria, this balloon in the area of your cheeks fills with fluid. The fluid increases the pressure, and gravity assists in the downward pressure right on the tip (apex) of the tooth, where the nerve supply is restricted. Sometime this is the cause of a toothache. If the teeth are hurting give yourself a little push on the cheek; apply pressure to the cheek bones in the area just below the eye. If this increases the discomfort on your teeth, wait to call the dentist until the sinuses are less aggravated. Now, don't blame the sinuses if it has been hurting for weeks.

The fifth trigeminal nerve comes out of the neck and provides muscular movement. It also supplies the bulk of the nerve activity to a large area of the face. Sometimes you will have an earache, and the source will really be a problem with a tooth (wisdom teeth are notorious). It is possible for the problem to be with a top tooth, while discomfort manifests itself in the lower jaw. All of us are wired differently. There is a general standard of route that a nerve will take in most people, but you just might be special. Wisdom teeth (third molars) are able to position themselves in areas where they can take you to your knees with discomfort, by applying pressure on this nerve supply.

Sinus Drainage

Wait until your sinuses are better before you blame your teeth for that pressure pain. The roots of your teeth meet or extend into the maxillary sinus cavities. Pressure of sinuses caused by the drainage is what is coming out of your nose and down your throat. That pressure also strains the blood supply trying to get to the tooth's nerve canal. The nerve of the tooth communicates this pain. Apply pressure to the cheeks. If this makes the teeth hurt more, it just might be the sinuses.

Rinse out your sinuses with a Neti pot, which you can get at your local drug store. It's a little pot or bulb that you fill with saline. You lay your head sideways over the sink, and pour the saline into your upper nostril (or squeeze the bulb). The saline trickles through your nasal system and comes out your other nostril. It sounds as if it might hurt, but it doesn't. Saline has a similar make-up as your own fluids, and if it's warm, it feels easy and natural. This will give you relief by flooding your sinuses gently with saline to wash them out more completely, quicker and safer than a run to the doctor for a prescription.

Sinus pain can also result in similar discomfort during altitude changes. Airplanes and scuba diving change the amount of pressure, resulting in a difference in the external and internal body pressure. Discomfort commonly resides when one returns to the altitude one normal lives under.

Tori (Extra Boney Area Around The Jaw)

These are extra boney growths on either arch of the mouth. A torus is a non-pathological outgrowth of bone (no disease). Some believe these exostoses (extra one) are genetically linked; others think they occur because of behavioral practices, possibly a result of stressful habits (biting nails or other objects, grinding and clenching of teeth).

Do you have a hard boney bump under your tongue? If you hit it with your toothbrush, do you almost want to cry? If the toothbrush does hit the area, does it become an ulcer within hours? That is a TORUS.

Why do these form? Recent thought is, "IT JUST HAPPENS."

Sometimes during the formation of the jawbone, the bone just forgets to stop forming and this growth of extra bone is developed. If you think wearing a denture will be easy, try placing a basketball under a saddle of a horse and going for a pleasure ride. WRONG.

Sometimes during the changes of life- people in the fifty to sixty year age group- for some reason this boney development will start forming again. Bone is breaking down everywhere else in the body, but in the mouth, bone can get overgrown. In my years of working the dental field, I have seen people so affected by this, that the shape of their faces was changed by the development of this boney growth. Some had this bone surgically removed and did fine. Sometimes the growth was back in full force within a year.

Gum Recession

Gum recession occurs when tissue tightens with age and moves down the tooth. Skin tightens in the mouth as we age. The tooth is designed like a funnel. As the tissue tightens, it will move down the tooth and expose new portion of the tooth, the root surface. All of us will have it to some degree. Some of us will have pain such as with a toothache.

Steps that can be followed at home that cost less and just might work are:

First: Refrain from rinsing out your toothpaste. Fluoride is the best treatment to cover these exposed dentin tubules, as long as there is a good source of calcium in your diet.

Second: Ask the pharmacist for a fluoride. It is behind the counter, comes in many flavors, and contains just a higher percentage of fluoride (Fl2). You should keep it away from children, because the flavors may make them think it is candy. It could make them vomit. Remember, it is for the teeth not the stomach. Keep in mind that you must select the type of fluoride that works with you. (Reviewed in toothpaste section)

Third: There are treatments that cost in the fifty-dollar range, feel sticky and taste bad, but they work great. (Varnish) A hygienic form of varnish is the chemical used in the dental office. It works simply by reducing the nerve's exposure to the changing environment in the mouth. You can spit out the extra, but there seems to be no problem with swallowing.

Research has shown that fluoride is needed throughout life because gum recession extends the cavity stage. With fresh parts of the tooth exposed to the environment of the mouth at different times, chemicals need to be present to fortify.

Cold-Sensitive Teeth

Welcome to a birthday gift you get and didn't ask for. The tissue in your mouth will tighten with age. The tooth is built like a funnel, large on top and smaller where it meets the gum. When these areas of the tooth are exposed, you can feel a chill. The teeth have grown accustomed to having a 98 degree blanket on them. They tend to complain when that's gone. The temperature and PH changes in the mouth are not comfortable. They cannot tell they are just feeling Rocky Road ice cream or a fresh bite of orange.

The root portion (dentin) is half as strong as the top of the tooth (enamel), and the body has a built-in, self-protective design. Small holes are on this part (dentin), and tiny nerve endings are present in the caverns. So, if decay does occur, the response is quick. Discomfort will occur when there is direct communication between the internal nerve and blood supply to the outside world. This nerve only speaks one language: pain. It cannot speak about pressure, temperature or PH.

There is an area where the tooth meets the gum called the CEJ (Cemento-Enamel Junction). In this area of the tooth structure lies a great area of controversy. Maybe you are one of those people who can take a finger nail and find a dent in the body of the tooth where the tooth meets the tissue (pink stuff). This broken area is called many names.. Was it caused by brushing your teeth as if they were the grill on the BBQ pit, causing abrasions? Maybe. Or was it caused by the bending of the tooth because of force placed on the top (the chewing surface) by moving the tooth in the wrong direction, causing abfraction?

The tooth is built like a heart, with its chewing surface in the top of the heart and the pointed tip leading down to the root. When force is placed on the surface of the tooth, pressure is built up internally. To compensate, the tooth will flex and rock in an outward bend at the gum line (CEJ). This flex will slowly cause bits of the tooth to pop off causing sensitivity and "dents" at the gum line. Abfraction is the result of the bending. There are many reports to support both as a cause. The material used to repair these is the same as for cavities. It is done by placing tooth-colored chemicals to fill the V-shape defect, but the hole has to be deep enough for the filler to hold on during regular tooth functions. In some cases you might have to wait until the hole gets bigger (that's a strange thought), so the material will not pop out or be brushed out of position.

Grafts

Grafts can be attached to replace gingival (gums) lost for a multiple of reasons. Tissue is obtained from donors and is treated to ensure its safety, or you can have it harvested from the roof of your mouth. Yes, creating an area that will feel like the pizza burn that rewarded you when you failed to wait for the food to cool down. You will be provided with a plastic shield to cover the roof of the mouth until it heals. The area where the tissue is placed will have little or no discomfort. Since the body recognizes the tissue, a compatible blood supply will be provided by the surrounding tissue. Grafts are a must if there is a loss of too much of the attached gingival flesh (pink gums). There are two types of tissue in the mouth. One is like the palm of the hand (attached: strong work hardy surface) and the other is like the top of your hand (unattached: loose movable tissue).

The front teeth are under continuous attack by the tongue. The tongue is the strongest muscle in the body, even stronger than the heart. With every swallow the tongue hammers up to the front teeth and then pushes the elements on the tongue backward, unless you have a reverse swallow. Then the tongue pushes itself out and up. This will cause you to stick out your tongue and often hold it out in your relaxed position. This is called a reverse swallow.

With so much pressure being applied to the teeth, the reason they do not drift forward is because of the muscles in the lips and this attached gingival (gums). Pull out your lips and wiggle them a bit. See the difference between the attached and unattached gingival (pink tissue). The teeth need both to hold position; lose attached tissue and the tooth will drift forward from the hammering of the tongue. Don't think the new surgically placed tissue will have the strength to push the tooth back. It will only reduce future movement. Movement of teeth happens with braces.

We are born with a set quantity of mouth tissue. This tissue is very sophisticated and cannot be reproduced by the body in quantity, except on the roof of the mouth. It is like cutting off a finger, the tip never grows back.

If the teeth are very crowded, and a lot of movement during braces has to occur, sometimes there is not enough tissue to cover all the newly arranged teeth. This is where a graft becomes the perfect solution. Also if you brush your teeth as if you are cleaning the B-B-Q pit, you might be discussing grafts with the surgeon in the future.

Grinding Or Clenching Teeth

Have you ever watched someone's facial muscles move but they were not talking. They are working the teeth on overtime, with nothing in between, to prevent them from working on each other. The masseter muscle, which helps us talk, chew, and open and closes the jaw, is being abused during this over active time of grinding and/or clenching.

Think of it as if you were lifting weights. Have you ever seen a mechanic or weight lifter who has lost the ability to extend his arm out all the way, and has lost his range of motion? All day, as mechanics are turning wrenches, they don't stop to extend the arm out into a relaxed position. Slowly, the muscles will change what they consider a relaxed position. This goes for facial muscles. They are exercised while eating, talking, chewing gum, biting your nails, etc. It is not considered a habit to stop, and stretch the muscle (yes a muscle) back into a relaxed position, just like after any exercise. They are called facial muscles! Think of an athlete who will warm up, work the muscles, and stretch the muscle back to the normal working position to prevent injury.

Facial muscles have the ability to crack pecans during waking hours, with a full range of motion of about one to two inches of opening. By decreasing the starting point and increasing the strength that is applied, the result is costly to you. Fractured teeth are pieces of bone with a nerve supply in the middle, sawing back and forth across this nerve. This thought should make your skin crawl.

Teeth inserted into the jawbone are like lacing your straight finger together.

The right hand would be the teeth and the left hand the jaw bone. In this intersection there is padding, as there is with every bone in the body

It's called a periodontal ligament. (Perio means mouth.) The ligament here is no different than anywhere else in the body, such as the elbow or knee, except, that at the end of the tooth there is the blood and nerve supply entering into the tooth. When the right hands fingers is hammered into the left's hands fingers, as during grinding or clenching, the effect is like a stone bruise. With your foot, you can avoid the painful area and try not to apply pressure on the site for a day or week. You can try chewing on the other side, but the teeth will all meet with every chew. Keep up the hammering on a bruised area and the side effect is destructive. Trauma of the teeth can come from the area of the periodontal ligament (shock absorbers). Let's call it a runaway stone bruise.

Just ask my face, it hit the bottom of a swimming pool at the age of 12 after jumping off the low board of a small apartment complex pool. The impact of the unbroken tooth was forced into the surrounding bone support. Ten years later a dime size void was detected in x-rays. Then came Root canal, Reroot canal, Apico (cut off root tip), Re-Apico and a half a dozen crowns later, I still have my smile.

One patient was x-rayed and the x-rays showed no bone in the chin. They said they could remember going down to pick up their child, just as the child jumped up. "My chin was sore and bruised; I thought that it would just heal." They were lucky; six root canals later, the bone started regenerating. Left untreated, if the area had received another impact, a surgical reconstruction of the chin with the assistance of a portion of the hip bone might have been necessary.

Now, I would call that a runaway bruise!

Tmd Or Tmj - Temporal Mandibular Dysfunction Or Junction

Temporal bones and muscles are located just in front of the ears and fan out and upwards like opening your fingers and extending them up to the sky. The Mandibular bone connects in front of the ear, forms an 'L' shape, and carries the teeth in the lower jaw and provides the motion for eating and talking. Dysfunction happens when these areas do not play together nicely, or is overworked by the bad habits listed below. The facial muscles were designed for eating only, not for all the other habits modern mankind has added to the day's events.

Bad habits are: Sleeping with your hand up around the face
Chewing gum
Biting your fingernails
Chewing on your cheek, lips or tongue
Resting your head on our shoulder
    when holding the phone
Snacking on beef jerky or carrots too often
Cracking pecans with our teeth
Holding objects in our teeth, such as
    pins, nails, fishing wire, etc.
Opening the mouth to wide and
    hearing a pop or click

Clicking and Popping in the ear is not a normal or good sound to hear, that's bone on bone. Nature provided us with a cushion to comfort the rotation of movement. In the jaw area it is more like a pillow. There is nowhere else in the body with a movement or design of structure more elegant than the TMJ area.

The masseter muscle is attached to the cheek bone, and extends to the jaw bone. Some recent research is looking into the possibility that this facial design might have been the turning point in the shape and size of the human brain. It is under consideration that the tension change of this muscle might have led to enlargement of the brain. Yes, I watch Nova on **PBS**.

When the masseter muscle is overworked and shortened from the building of the muscle and the lack of stretching the muscle, something has to give. In structural design the next muscle up the chain is called upon to make up for the need of function. This is the temporal muscle. Weeks and months go by and the range of motion of this muscle is reduced. Next. If this continues over a years, the shoulders and mid back can be affected, and change from having to make movements that the over-worked, shortened masseter muscles just could not perform.

Just touch someone with this condition on the top of the shoulder, midway to the neck and ever so slightly to the back. You might want to stand back, because they might take a swing at you. Ask them if it feels like a knife in the back, sometime hot then painfully stone cold. Ask if the shoulder jerks up at times unexpectedly.

You can see why, with so much muscle contraction happening to the bone surrounding the brain, that this might be the cause of your headaches, or neck and back discomfort.

TMJ or TMD @ help guide.org

@WebMD.org   (many, many other web sites)

Treatment For Tmj

Braces and/or Mouth pieces can assist in the pain reduction.

CURING IS A PROBLEM

Help is possible and with it a great improvement in relief of pain. Stress is the leading cause of grinding or clenching. Just take those problems to bed and work them out in your mind, and as you fall asleep just keep working on them with your facial muscles. Females might have a greater percentage of occurrences then men because of the hormone differences.

Common response to enquiries is,

"I just don't think I do either of those things, I am almost sure!" Then take a quick test:

In that, conversation-slash argument, just stop a minute and ask yourself,

"WHAT ARE MY TEETH DOING?"

When you are running late, and/or traffic is backed up, ask yourself,

"WHAT IS MY JAW DOING?"

Ask your sleeping partner,

"Do I sound like I am eating rocks at night?"

GOOD HABIT: KEEP LIPS TOGETHER
BUT TEETH APART

You people lifting weights, please, place a mouth guard or something between your teeth when you slam your teeth together during the heavy lift. " O, is that the reason a part of my tooth fell off! "

Snoring And Sleep Apnea

**THIS MUST BE DISCUSSED WITH
YOUR MEDICAL DOCTOR FIRST**

The obstruction of the airway can cause snoring. Blow through a straw. If you want to make a noise, squeeze it in the middle. That is how snoring happens. In the throat there are many things that can obstruct the flow of air. Here are a few:

First, open your mouth. Can you see your tonsils?
Or is your tongue in the way (to big)
Second, look again. Are the tonsils kissing?
Is this where the straw is squeezed shut?
Third, if you can't swallow pills, **how can air move
through when the chin falls back while
sleeping on your back?** This is why rolling
a person over makes them stop snoring!
Fourth, the weight of your chest and neck need to
be considered because of weight/pressure.
Is it a thick barrel type?

APNEA is when you stop breathing for minutes during the night. Many studies are out that agree that this breathing function will take years off your life. The heart will increase your blood pressure when you have a breathing malfunction. Your lungs will spasm, trying to return to rhythm. With so many natural body functions going haywire, good sleep will not occur. Your mind needs to wake you up to assist in basic breathing habits. Ask yourself, "Do I dream?" Dreams happen in REM (rapid eye movement) sleep. You can't stay asleep long enough to enter REM sleep with some of these bodily mishaps.

Your dentist has a mouthpiece that can be worn to reposition the lower jaw DOWN AND FORWARD, allowing an enlarging of the opening from the lips to the lungs. First, the necessary tests need to be completed by your medical doctor, to prove the presents of Apnea. Then C-Pap; a breathing machine will be discussed and reviewed for home use, that sounds like a 747 blasting off in your bedroom, and the mask was no doubt copied from Darth Vader, with duplication of his sounds effects. High forces of pressurized air apply by this devise, will force the airway open. This is the reason for the noise and the mask. These tests must be completed and a trial of the C-Pap will need to occur, before the dentist can discuss the Snoring apparatus, that will position the lower jaw down and forward, opening the airway.

Apnea Must Be Discuss with Your Medical Doctor FIRST

This is a book about common sense dentistry, not a diagnosis. Agree; some people have difficulty wearing oral objects over night. Remember this is a mouthpiece that is a superman version of a football mouth guard, can be obtained at your dentist of record. With No drugs, and very light side effects, you just might return to a good night's sleep and dreaming.

Can't say I have seen the one advertised on television.

Sleep apnea can be the leading cause of many major health problems.

Sleep apnea@helpguide.org

@Web MD.org   (many, many other web sites)

This is a book of Common Sense Dentistry

**SOMEONE ASK ME IF IT REALLY MADE ME MAD THAT
SOME PEOPLE DO NOT TAKE CARE OF THEIR TEETH
NOPE: JOB SECURITY**

This is a book about Common Sense Dentistry

Not a diagnosis

**Visit your dentist twice a year for an exam
As the birthdays add up, make it three or four times**

**Promise the over all bills will be <u>LESS</u>
Along with your <u>pain</u> and <u>lost minutes</u> of life and work**

SPECIALIST often referrals, made by your dentist

PEDODONTIST — Specialize in the care of children
    Zero to eighteen years

ORTHODONTIST — Working with the jaw alignment and
    Arrangement of the teeth (Braces)

ORAL SURGEON — Specialize in the removal or repair
    of the area below the nose and to the
    chin Implants can be discussed

PERIODONTIST — Working with the soft tissue surrounding
    the teeth also Implants

PROSTODONTIST — Specializing in the replacement of
    Missing teeth
    (Dentures, Partials and Implants)

OTOLARYNGOLOGY — Ears, Nose and Throat
(ENT)

Products   I Like

Biotene moisturizing
Gel or Spray –   enzymes needed in mouth

Dentex Easy Angle
Flossers –   handy flossers for back teeth

Proxbrushes –   help remove larger food particles between teeth

Soft toothbrushes – No other texture for the mouth

Small headed
toothbrushes –   take care of teeth individually: please

Thorton Flossers – great for implants, bridges and braces (pink box my favorite)

Bridge Threaders – for braces, implants and crowns (if Thorton flossers can not be found)

Home Fluorides –   just ask the pharmacy
                   Does not take prescription
                   Use only if the mouth is very clean,
                   Don't rinse this out with water
                   It need to stay on the teeth

Glide Wax Floss –   just stronger and tears less

POH Unwaxed floss – only if you have been flossing
                       For Over 5 years
                       This will cut if handled wrong

Denture brushes –   for cleaning of all parts of dentures
                       Plastic and metal
                       Double sided it's a big brush
                       Never use in mouth

Act Home Fluoride
     for Children –   good for all ages
                       Apply with Q-tip if to young to spit

GUM WITH XYITOL–look for the ADA seal

**Please review the warning by the FDA on children's
TEETHING PRODUCTS**

Need help understanding your dental bill, there in a code

(Updates are made frequently)

ada.org/codes (type in the year)

ADA Dental Codes
(American Dental Association)
211 EAST CHICAGO AVE
CHICAGO IL. 60611-2678

www.ingramcontent.com/pod-product-compliance
Lightning Source LLC
Chambersburg PA
CBHW051330170526
45166CB00002B/755